Breema ~ Essence of Harmonious Life

Other books from
California Health Publications

Touching the Mountain — The Self-Breema Handbook:
Ancient Exercises for the Modern World

Flame of the Uncharted Heart: Essential Poetry

Song of the Uncharted Heart: Essential Poetry

Dance of the Uncharted Heart: Essential Poetry

———————

Design and production assistance by
Sharyn Venit, Taos Mountain Press, Santa Fe, NM

Photography by George Draper
Berkeley, CA

Front and back cover photography by Galen Rowell
Mountain Light Photography
Berkeley, CA

Breema ~ Essence of Harmonious Life

by Jon Schreiber

California Health Publications
Oakland, California

California Health Publications
6201 Florio Street, Suite 1A
Oakland, CA 94618

510-428-1283

fax 510-428-2705

www.breema.com

ISBN: 0–9623581–7-7

Library of Congress Catalog Card Number: 97-069542

Printed in the United States of America

Breema℠–Breema is a service mark of the Breema Center

Printed on recycled paper

Real health means one thing:
harmony with Existence.

Jon Schreiber

Jon Schreiber is director of the Breema Center and of the Advanced Arts Breema Chiropractic Clinic in Oakland, California. Dr. Schreiber prepared for a traditional medical degree at Columbia University in New York and subsequently became interested in alternative approaches to health and healing. Concurrent with receiving his chiropractic degree from Palmer College of Chiropractic–West, he was introduced to Breema bodywork. Finding the Breema method unique in its ability to vitalize and heal the body, Dr. Schreiber has devoted many years to studying and teaching this system. Besides caring for patients in his clinic, he maintains an active teaching schedule both nationally and internationally.

He has also devoted great energy to documenting various aspects of this unwritten tradition. His first book, *Touching the Mountain*, is an illustrated guide for doing Self-Breema exercises. *Flame of the Uncharted Heart, Song of the Uncharted Heart,* and *Dance of the Uncharted Heart* are a three-volume series of original poetry, collected and revised by Dr. Schreiber. Dr. Schreiber lives in Oakland, California with his wife Dana and their two children.

Author's Note

I am grateful to sixteen years of study of *All and Everything* and *Meetings with Remarkable Men*, written by Gurdjieff himself, and to my study with the students of Gurdjieff's students. *Breema - Essence of Harmonious Life* is written with the insight I received from my work with the Gurdjieff Teaching.

For those who have an interest in Gurdjieff, I recommend reading *All and Everything* (*Beelzebub's Tales to His Grandson - An Objectively Impartial Criticism of the Life of Man*) and *Meetings with Remarkable Men*.

Acknowledgments

The material presented in this book was collected from tape recordings and transcriptions of Breema classes taught between 1980 and 1997 at the Breema Center. Malichek Mooshan was born and grew up in the village of Breema, and is the first person to teach Breema outside of the village. Additional material was excerpted from my notes of many meetings and conversations with Malichek over the years. Malichek personally reviewed every sentence of the final manuscript and worked with me until he was satisfied that it conveyed the essence of the Breema method and its principles and philosophy accurately.

Many other people contributed tremendous time and energy to help create this book:

Susan Varner lent support in many ways.

Gretchen Brandt organized, edited, researched information from the Breema Center's archives, and coordinated the design, production, photography, and printing of the book.

Special thanks to those instructors at the Center who appear in the photographs—Marian Clark, Mary Cuneo, Ashik Staud, Denise Berezonsky, Ann Hudson, Gretchen Brandt, Celeste McLean and Arlie Mischeaux.

David Curry worked hard on an earlier draft of the Breema book, as did Sharyn Venit. Sharyn also collaborated on typesetting and design, and handled the page layout and production. Gwynne Hooke cheerfully typed and retyped and retyped the manuscript. Lisa Schiffman helped edit early versions of the book. Peter Hensel generously made available the class notes he compiled over more than a decade. Editorial help was also provided by Marian Clark, Gretchen Brandt, Ashik Staud, Denise Berezonsky, Christine Hunt, and Jan Winitz.

Sandy Taylor, The Graphic Page, helped with the cover design.

Thanks to the Breema Center's first staff group: Caite Bennett, David Bierman, Nancy Crum,

Ayumie Kie, Eddie Bauman, and Ann Cummings. Thanks are also due to everyone who has worked over the years to create and maintain the archives of the Breema Center, and to the Center's current staff and to the students whose interest, participation, and questions created a need for this material to be presented.

Thanks to my wife, Dana, for her constant support and for everything she did in order to make time for me to work on this book.

For their support, I also thank: Janet Madden, Aron Saltiel, Pari Schneider, Janet Chann, Evan Specter, Roxanna O'Leary, Susan Patton, Lauren Kline, Shannon Schroter, Elaine Pendergrast, Jean Haseltine, Steve Pendergrast, Joy Rowan, Bruce Barrett, Robin Somerville, Michael Irwin, Sally Riedman, Don Cohen, Rebecca Spalten, Tatjana Kopp, Ann Hudson, Jon Lobdell, Alexandra Sheets, Roxanne Schroter, Alicia Carter, Mike Reid, Gerrie Leach, Avishai Pearlson, T'Shala Vahsen, Claudia Saltiel, Lauren Varner-Movlai, Amanda Movlai, Sophie Staud, Sarita Flor Schreiber, Noah Amir Schreiber, and Rafael.

Disclaimer

Breema was developed by people who had profound insight into the structure and function of the human body, and its relationship to the four levels of Existence: matter, energy, Consciousness, and Awareness. The bodywork and exercises are an expression of the natural and Universal laws which govern the body and its health. The reader must carefully employ the principles underlying the treatments, using caution and common sense whenever attempting to practice any of the treatments outlined in the book.

This book is for educational purposes and is designed to familiarize the reader with basic principles of Breema. It is sold with the understanding that the publisher and author are not engaged in rendering medical or other professional health service via the book and its contents. The reader must clearly understand that Breema bodywork, including the treatments presented in Part II, can only be properly learned in a live setting, from a Certified Breema Instructor. This book is not intended as a substitute for classroom training in Breema bodywork. In order to become a Breema Practitioner, completion of the Breema Center Certification Program is required. Consult a health professional if you have questions or problems. The author and publisher shall have neither liability nor responsibility to any person or entity with respect to any loss, damage, or injury caused or alleged to be caused directly or indirectly by the information contained in this book.

I am very happy to see the philosophy, principles, and method of Breema so accurately communicated on paper. This is an authentic presentation of Breema—a practical, unmanipulated method derived from the wisdom of the Earth, the natural laws governing life, and an understanding of the Timeless nature of Existence.

I'm deeply grateful to Dr. Jon Schreiber, Gretchen Brandt, Marian Clark, Jan Winitz, Denise Berezonsky, Janet Madden, Pari Schneider, Aron and Claudia Saltiel, Mary Cuneo, Ann Hudson, and to all instructors of Breema for their help and dedication in bringing Breema to many people's lives.

As you do Breema, let the joy of Existence be present with you. Be as simple as you can be. There is no need for activity in your mind and feelings. Drop all expectation. And if you need to occupy your mind, just registering the weight of the body and the fact of inhalation and exhalation will do.

Malichek Mooshan

To the heart.
To the Truth that is in the heart.
To the heart that is Existence itself.
That which is not Love is fatal.

TABLE OF CONTENTS

APPENDICES

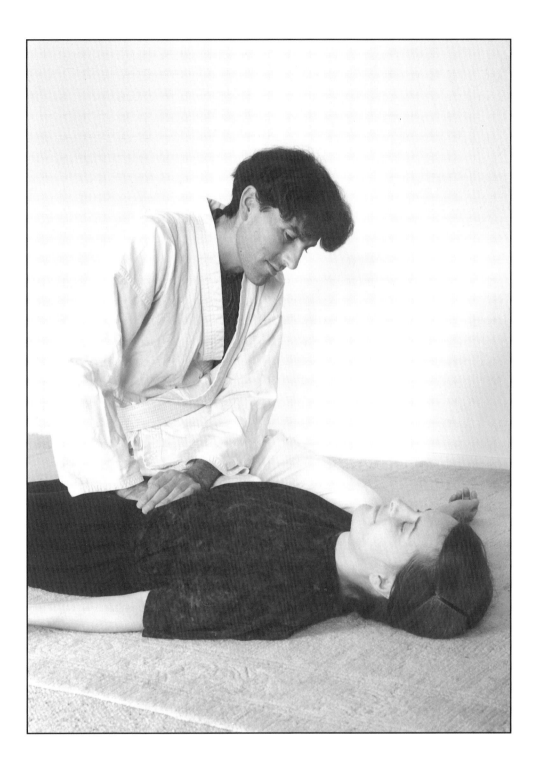

PREFACE

One of my earliest memories is of standing up in my bed when I was very little, dancing to a jingle on the radio. The natural joy of being alive and the equally natural expression of that joy later turned out to be rather elusive things. In retrospect, I see that the search for them has been the motivating force in my life.

As a child, I loved the aliveness of gypsy and ethnic folk music. I studied classical violin for ten years, six of them at Juilliard, but the rigid training lacked the spark I was looking for.

Science had always appealed to me because of the promise it held of hope for humanity, and so I decided to study medicine because it seemed the most human and interactive branch of science. I prepared for medical school at Columbia University, studied biology at the Hebrew University in Jerusalem, and behavioral science at Oberlin College. But no matter where I studied, I was unable to escape the disillusionment I felt with the mechanistic, material approach to the body.

After university, I moved to Ann Arbor, where, because of a back injury, I found myself for the first time visiting a chiropractor. Dr. Bobby Rose was dedicated and intelligent, and his enthusiasm for the profession led me to enroll in chiropractic school two years later. I had high hopes of learning a natural, drug-less healing system, but instead found myself immersed in studying anatomy, physiology, and pathophysiology from morning until night.

While in school in California, a friend told me about a man who was teaching a wonderful method of bodywork in Berkeley. I went to an evening open house to see it.

Although his English was ungrammatical and heavily accented, Malichek Mooshan (the man who was presenting Breema) spoke with disarming simplicity, and with a naturalness I'd never heard before. His words made sense without trying to convince — they simply illuminated the subject of health and the body. When he asked for a volunteer and began giving a Breema treatment, I immediately realized I had stumbled onto something magical. The earthy beauty of the treatment's movements and its natural rhythm and grace created a riveting atmosphere that was unlike anything I had seen or experienced before. I knew I had to study it. I made an appointment for my girlfriend to get a treatment, hoping she'd take a Breema class together with me.

I brought her to Malichek's apartment and, without questioning her at all, he asked her to lie down fully clothed on a Persian rug in his classroom, which was a virtual jungle of leafy house plants and trays of sprouts. His short treatment cleared her sinuses, which in itself was amazing — due to chronic allergies, they had always been blocked.

Then, he offered me a treatment. When he placed his hand on my chest, right over a bony indentation, he said only, "This you already know." His acknowledgment of this physical particularity was totally free of judgment, and in the simplest way, gave me my first taste of the deepest healing principle of Breema — acceptance.

Breema classes were a healing balm for me. Just watching the treatments being demonstrated was healing! The classes were practical — a treatment was shown, and then the students would pair up and practice it. Feedback was always based on actual experience. Whenever Malichek spoke, his words had a natural authority based on self-verified experience. He had a way of bringing things into clear focus for the mind, while speaking straight to the heart, often illustrating his subject with folk tales and parables. At the same time, he placed everything he spoke about in a greater context, always emphasizing the interrelatedness of things. I experienced a gradual reawakening of the desire to really understand my body, my life, and my relation to the Universe. The desire for truth, and the questions about life I had as a child, which, by the time I was in my teens, I had despaired of ever finding answers to, re-emerged and were nurtured by the atmosphere of total acceptance in the classes. Understanding was spoken of, not as a collection of concepts in the mind, but as something that could be *received* when one creates an *inner authority,* a *Being.*

The classes had an atmosphere of tremendous vitality and aliveness that gave me a tangible feeling of health and well-being. In addition to the essential psychological and emotional balancing that Breema provided, it was also helping to dissolve my body's crystallizations. I had grown up with an incredibly stiff, inflexible body, and from early childhood, my repertoire of comfortable postures was very limited. Sitting on the floor had always been extremely uncomfortable.

Thanks to Breema, I found myself becoming more flexible. Breema is ground (floor) based, and the transition from chair to floor, though at first difficult for me, had a revolutionary effect on my health.

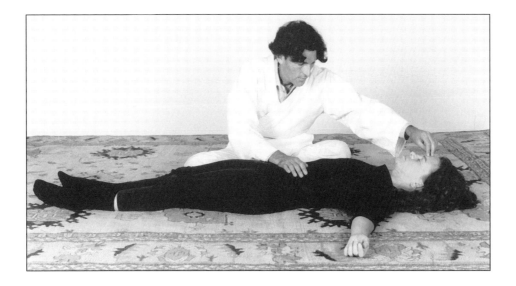

My initial enthusiasm and perseverance in practicing Breema quickly started to pay off. In classes, because I was always the stiffest, I had the most difficulty doing the treatments. So at night, I'd call up my friends, pestering them to let me practice the "latest" sequences on them. After a few weeks, the pattern was reversed; people began calling *me*.

During the day at chiropractic school, I learned specific adjusting techniques, credited to one of chiropractic's founding fathers. But, amazingly enough, at night in Breema class, treatment sequences were often presented that allowed the body to make the same adjustments itself, without sacrificing any of the Breema principles.

The turning point in my relationship to Breema came after a bad fall dislocated two of my ribs. For a whole month, I couldn't inhale without sharp pain. Nothing I tried seemed to help. Finally, I made an appointment to get a treatment from Malichek, not mentioning my problem.

Without posing any questions, Malichek asked me to lie down. He gave me a short treatment, working gently, and only on my legs. It was pleasant, and seemingly unremarkable. He bowed and left the room. I remember my first feeling was relief at finding the pain was still there. This was a secret test I had set for Breema, actually hoping it would fail! After investing so many years in both medical and chiropractic study, I wasn't yet ready to acknowledge the profound efficacy of this down-to-earth method. Ten minutes later, though, I found the area of rib pain shrinking, the way the circle of light shrinks on an old television set when you shut it off. In minutes, the pain disappeared completely, and never came back.

The words used so often in Breema class had a new meaning for me:

There is only one body, and no matter where you touch, you're touching the whole body.
The body is Universal. It functions with the principle of inner connectedness.
Every cell is blessed with total knowledge of the whole, and so is always in unity with it.

Now I understood how, by working on my legs, Breema helped my ribs heal. I began taking it more seriously.

By the time I entered the school clinic as a student doctor, I knew I wanted to practice Breema. My patients loved it and asked for more.

Between patient appointments, I shed my white clinic uniform and practiced Breema treatments on the soccer field out back. There was always a line of eager recipients that eventually included several of the more open-minded faculty members, who became "regulars."

After graduating, I opened my practice, constantly adapting and refining chiropractic technique by applying the principles of Breema to it. I soon stopped using an adjusting table, and did all my chiropractic work on a rug — Breema style.

Every patient visit included Breema bodywork, and I started to prescribe Self-Breema exercises therapeutically. I was receiving incredibly positive feedback, and my practice kept growing. I moved it to a bigger office and hired several Breema practitioners to assist me.

Teaching the principles of Breema to my patients was natural and necessary, and allowed them to take an active part in their own recovery and health maintenance. Studying Breema took on an added dimension for me — I was there not only to learn Breema, but also to learn how to best teach it.

Over the years I've been very fortunate in seeing Breema help thousands of patients and students through a great variety of health problems, as well as in watching them gain in ability to respond and adapt successfully to many difficult life situations by working with its principles. My respect for it only grows deeper, and I've found that its simplest beginning principles continue to unfold and deepen.

Because I had so often seen the simplest treatments, exercises, and principles exert such a transformative effect on people, it seemed natural to become involved in the administration of the Breema Center, and in teaching and writing about Breema. With the help of other dedicated students, I've had the privilege of helping the Center establish Breema Practitioner Certification programs in the United States and Europe, and an Instructor Certification program here in Oakland, California.

Now in my forties, I find my body healthier and more flexible than it was twenty years ago. I'm more active, but need less rest than I used to. Yet these are merely side effects, the "small magic" of Breema. Its real magic is that it enables us to experience the fact that "we are not what we think we are." Breema helps us let go of our conceptual body, and gives us a taste of our physiological body as a living phenomenon whose vitality is a function of the degree of harmony with the life force energy both inside and outside of it. It also gives us a way to unify our body, mind, and feelings in a common activity, which is the first step towards creating an inner authority that can have real understanding of our true nature and essential unity with Existence.

Jon Schreiber
Oakland, 1998

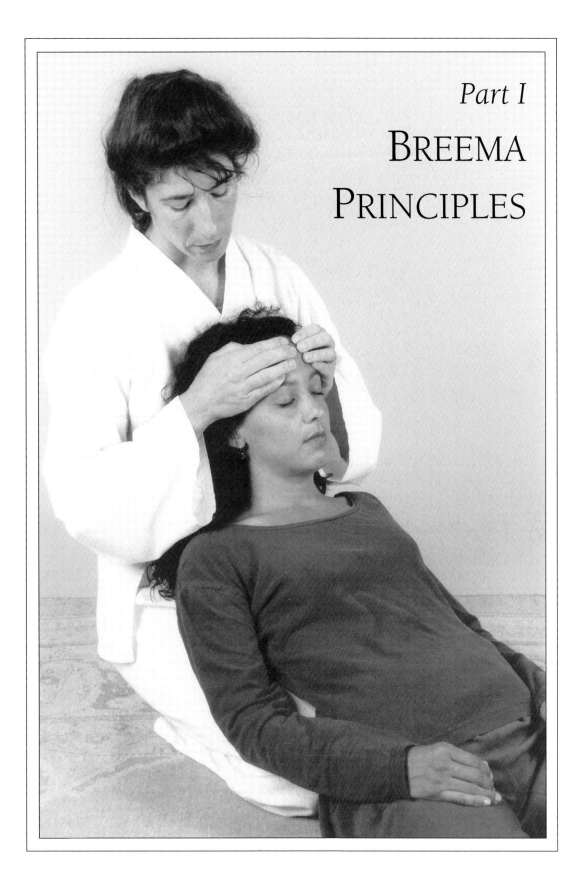

Part I

BREEMA
PRINCIPLES

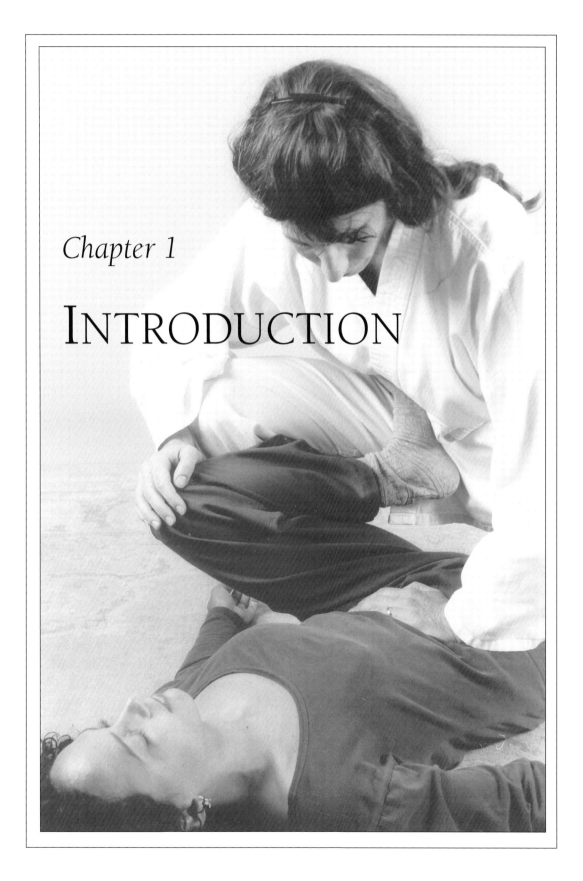

Chapter 1

INTRODUCTION

*"There is one Awareness, one Consciousness, one energy, **one** Existence. If you don't hear this in everything I say, you're not hearing me yet!"*

— Malichek Mooshan

INTRODUCTION

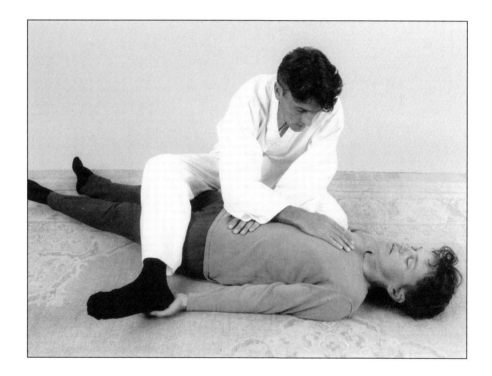

For years, people have been asking for a book presenting Breema's principles and philosophy. Although profoundly simple and completely natural, Breema is, in its nature, Universal.

The Breema Center has taught hundreds of treatment sequences and Self-Breema exercises in their exact form to students over the past eighteen years, yet these represent only a portion of the vast and varied repertoire of Breema. While certain aspects of Breema's principles and philosophy are beyond the scope of this book, the core of teachings of Breema are presented here.

Many people today recognize the need to access and understand the natural laws that govern human life and health, laws that offer a means of living in harmony with one's body, mind, and feelings, and with other people, the planet, and the Universe. It is fortuitous that just now, at the end of the twentieth century, Breema is starting to be taught and practiced in many different places. Through deep receptivity to the body, and a rhythmic connection to the Earth, Breema can help us become available to the instinctive wisdom of the body. By allowing that wisdom to participate with us in our daily lives, we can experience bountiful health and vitality. Breema enables us to benefit from the guidance that conection to the body offers in living a harmonious life and discovering its deeper meaning and purpose. In fact, connection to the body can serve as the initial impetus and support for our lifetime journey of self-discovery. This book was written with the aim of helping us take a step in that direction.

How to Benefit from this Book

Make sure your body is comfortable while you're reading. Relax. Breema is not something to be grasped by tense concentration. The first six chapters describe Breema principles and some general guidelines for practicing Breema. The photographs that accompany the text portray a wide variety of movements from many different Breema sequences. These pictures illustrate many of the Breema principles and can give you a visual taste of giving and receiving Breema. In Part II of the book, you'll find a photographic presentation of four treatment sequences. If you have never taken a class, you might want to skim through these treatments to get a visual impression of what Breema looks like before reading the book.

Some of the material will strike a resonant chord in you. Breema is based on a common-sense wisdom, so much of what you read may sound familiar, as if somehow you already knew it, even though you've never heard it said before. That's how Breema treatments are, too. Your body can learn them without tensing up because the movements are so natural they may feel like you've always known them, even though they're brand-new to you.

The principles are meant to be referred to again and again. As your experience and ability grow, so will your understanding. Don't hesitate to open the book to read a short section and let it sink in for awhile. Stay receptive as you read. Don't expect to comprehend everything at first glance. Don't settle with your first impression. Allow your relationship to Breema to ripen at a natural pace.

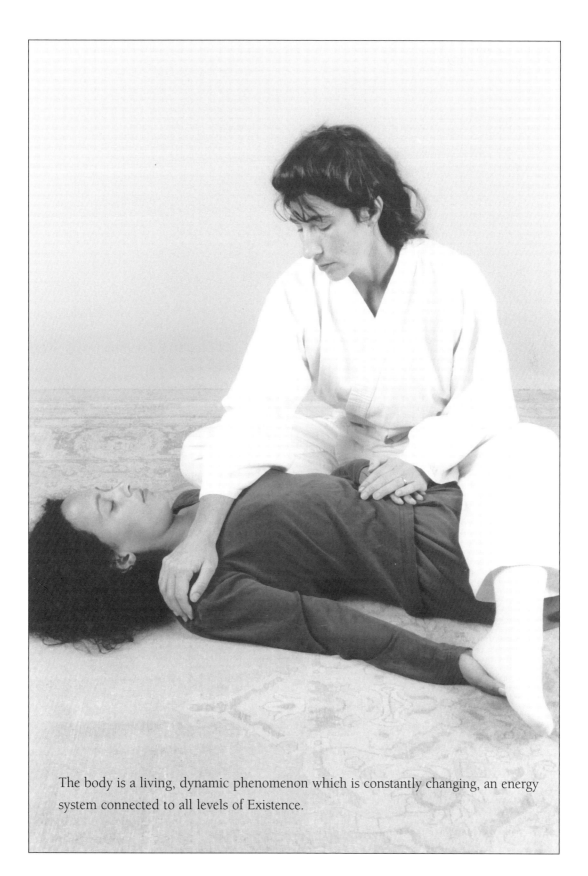

The body is a living, dynamic phenomenon which is constantly changing, an energy system connected to all levels of Existence.

It is wonderfully supportive for instructors and practitioners to read a couple of paragraphs in their classes or to their clients. The emanation of this book often helps create a receptive atmosphere.

If you want to study Breema, look for a Certified Breema Instructor in your area or come to study at the Breema Center (see Appendix). This book is just the beginning, just an appetizer. It may be delicious, but if you want to eat a real meal, you'll need to take a class. In class, you'll get the full range of tastes and experiences that can make Breema the most enjoyable and fulfilling study of your life.

A Brief Overview of the Breema Method — Its Principles and Philosophy

Breema is a method that slowly unfolds and deepens as one practices it. Its movements physically express the principles upon which they are based. These principles themselves are distilled from a profound understanding of the Universal Laws which govern life, and consequently, the body, its health, and its relationship to the energetic and physical aspects of the Universe. The philosophy of Breema is derived from these same laws. While, in its scope, it takes into consideration the four levels of Existence: matter, energy, Consciousness, and Awareness, and their interrelationships and essential unity, Breema is ultimately practical, and asks its students to take nothing on faith, but to accept as truth only that which they are able to verify for themselves.

What follows is a short orientation, so that as you read about Breema in subsequent chapters, you'll have a sense of how each principle relates to the whole. In fact, Breema is a truly hologenic system — each principle contains all the other principles within it. Every movement of each treatment sequence simultaneously calls for the application of all the principles, so by practicing any treatment, one can eventually discover every principle. This process of deepening our understanding is endless, and eventually can provide a definite direction for our lives, as we take a step towards self-understanding. The body is a laboratory in which we unite our mind, feelings, and physiology. When the unification of our three aspects is achieved, we have the possibility to realize our essential nature. We make understanding our own by living it.

The principles make Breema bodywork unique. They distinguish it from all other methods, even those which include movements that appear to be similar. Yet, the principles of Breema are Universal. They can be applied to other techniques and methods of bodywork, health improvement, health maintenance and, in fact, to any activity in life. Although, in this book, the principles are presented primarily in the context of the Breema bodywork method, they can be useful for everyone, not just for those who have an interest in bodywork. Readers will be able to extract enough clarity to begin, each in their own way, to apply those principles with which they find an inner resonance. If you find the principles inspiring, you will eventually want to support your study by participating in a class or workshop, because both practicing and receiving Breema bodywork is extremely helpful for deepening one's understanding.

The first principle of Breema is to make your body comfortable. This process starts even before you touch the recipient's body. Take a few breaths, and experience that your body is breathing, and that your body has weight on the ground. Almost immediately you can experience the refreshment of becoming available to yourself and to your immediate situation. Now, you're ready to touch your partner.

Many treatments begin with holding the instep/heel area of your partner's feet. According to the principle, you simply place your hands where they feel most comfortable to you. Your hands make complete contact as they gently mold to find a perfect fit with the contours of your partner's feet, without any tension. The practitioner constantly allows their own body to find a position of comfort and support, without compromise. Breema treatments require the body to assume many unique positions, yet are exactly suited to an experience of comfort for both practitioner and recipient.

Although simple, the principle of *body comfortable* is dynamic. By continually returning to your own body's comfort and the registration of your own weight and breathing, several beneficial things happen. Your energy is renewed and refreshed. As you practice, your body lets go of tension. You're allowing yourself the opportunity to fully participate in what you're doing. By focusing on the comfort of your own body, you're giving the recipient what their body needs, too. For example, when you lean your partner's legs towards their abdomen (see page 51), if their body is very flexible, it feels right to your body to lean in fully. But if your partner has some stiffness, you encounter resistance as you lean in, and your body amends the lean so it remains comfortable for both you and your partner. Breema doesn't use force. Your body leans in using only its natural weight, while at the same time supporting and stabilizing the recipient's body. Both bodies receive the security they need to release tension and to experience their natural state of vitality.

The principle of *using your whole body* is a natural correlate of *body comfortable*. The practitioner's every movement is made with the whole body, with "every single cell of the body participating." Some treatments require raising and rotating both of the recipient's legs or bringing the recipient from a supine to a sitting position. You can accomplish even these seemingly difficult movements without any tension or strain by using your whole body, instead of relying on the isolated muscular efforts of your arms or hands. All of its movements are made effortless, because **Breema doesn't ask the body to do anything that is not natural for it.** The body loves to do Breema movements, because you let your body stay comfortable and move with the whole body from your center of gravity.

The *knowing* that "I have a body" becomes the practitioner's center of balance and vitality. When you have this knowledge, you can do Breema simply, with the joy of full participation in your body's activity. Connection to the knowledge that "there is a body" is simple and natural, without anything "extra." It is not achieved through concentration, but by returning to the experience of your body's weight, breathing, and comfort.

When you receive a treatment, or if you watch someone doing Breema, you can experience and also see that the practitioner's hands are relaxed and free of tension, yet they touch without hesitation and always make full contact with the recipient. This is *"the Breema touch,"* which results from the principle of *firmness and gentleness*. Firmness comes from the registration of the relaxed weight of the body, while gentleness comes from the practitioner's presence and availability. We sometimes use the example of a mother holding her baby: the infant is securely, yet gently supported in her mother's arms.

The cornerstone principle of Breema is the *non-judgmental treatment*. Breema is non-diagnostic. Rather than focusing on the recipient, the emphasis is always on the experience of your own body. This non-judgmental approach includes the practitioner as well as the recipient, as both are supported to benefit from an atmosphere of acceptance. This principle says: "Don't try to fix anything. Don't fight sickness — increase vitality!" There is no need to impress others, and consequently no need for worry, anxiety, or criticism. While you give a treatment, you're doing the treatment for yourself. Nothing "extra" is needed. You can simply be alive and present. The atmosphere that is naturally created nurtures both giver and recipient, allowing them both to let go of tension and become vital and relaxed.

The Breema principles, applied in daily life, can make us free of the *conceptual* body — the ideas and images of our body that we carry in our mind. The conceptual body is divided into many separate parts — hands, arms, liver, legs, etc. We "see" these separate parts as

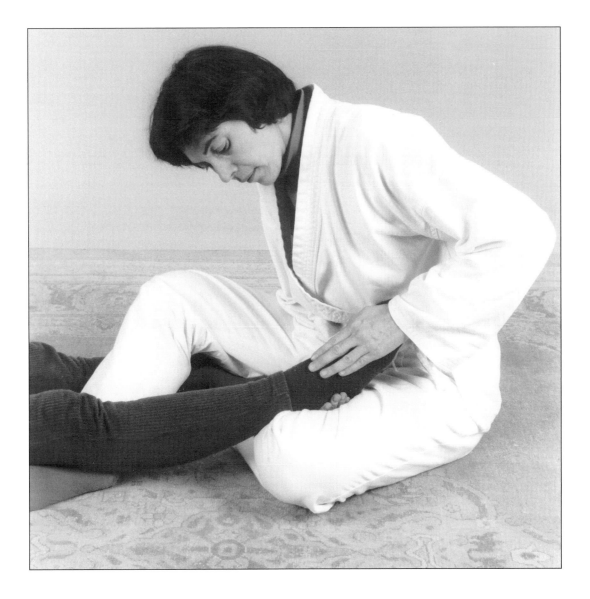

though they are distinct entities. We label them and identify with them. We forget they are part of a whole system. Breema encourages you to relate naturally to your physiological body — the body which you carry through life as a dynamic matter-energy combination. You become less and less subject to the ideas you've acquired about the body, and rely, instead, on your experience of your body.

In the same way, you are guided to discover the natural function of the mind — to receptively register the body's manifestations. This naturally functioning mind is very different from the mind we are accustomed to. The natural mind is receptive and available, and functions cooperatively with the body.

After your body and mind are balanced, it becomes possible for the feelings to function in their natural state. Instead of swinging between pleasant and unpleasant states, the feelings learn to be calm and balanced, lending a sense of supportive presence to the unified activity of the mind and body.

As a result, we function with our mind, body, and feelings in harmony, and we experience the unity of our three aspects. This unity serves as a foundation for the development of a unified Consciousness which can see things as they are.

Ultimately, Breema is more than a method. It is a natural, joyful, and harmonious response to Existence.

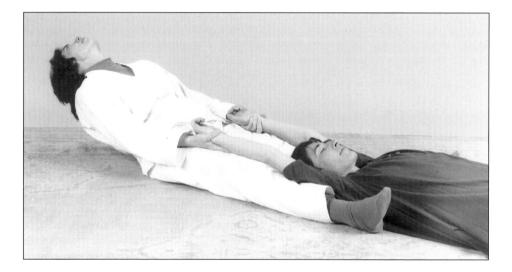

Existence consists of four levels: matter, energy, Consciousness, and Awareness itself.
Matter, energy, and Consciousness have no independent existence;
they are simply Awareness manifested.

Existence gives love to that which exists by simply expressing itself. On the human level, this love can be expressed through touch. In my village, the expression of touch through working on the body with stretches, leans, holds, and brushes was called Breema.

Breema is a Teaching of the heart, expressed in bodywork. Its purpose is to create harmony and balance for practitioner and recipient, and between Heaven and Earth.

In my village, my great grandfather was recognized as the principle Teacher of Breema in his time, and with tremendous love, care, and tenderness, he created conditions for the purpose of sharing his understanding with me. As my understanding of the meaning of my life in this body has grown, I've come to see that Breema is a wonderful medium for those who wish self-understanding. Greetings to all my friends who share this wish with me! Roll up your sleeves, and have fun being an expression of Existence.

—Malichek Mooshan

The Origin of Breema

Breema evolved in a remote mountain village in the Near East, and has been taught and practiced there since ancient times. All the villagers, including young children, practiced both partner treatments and Self-Breema exercises on a daily basis.

Breema was passed down through an unbroken lineage of Teachers. In each generation there was one such Teacher who had been specially trained by the previous Teacher. He or she was responsible for preserving the comprehensive body of treatments and exercises, for the "formal" instruction in Breema that everyone received beginning at age nine, and ultimately, for preparing the next Teacher. Neither the treatments nor the philosophy and principles of Breema were ever written down.

In the middle of the Nineteenth Century, a man whom the villagers called "Khan Baba" become the Teacher. He developed a very close relationship with his great grandson, Malichek Mooshan. Malichek learned Breema from Khan Baba, who took it upon himself to give Malichek a practical education in life by creating conditions in which he could share the depth of his understanding of life and of Breema principles, both in and out of the classroom. When Malichek was almost twenty years old, Khan Baba left this planet. Shortly afterward, Malichek left the village. Eventually coming to the West, Malichek became convinced of Breema's unique and enormous potential to benefit people living in modern society. He has worked ever since to create conditions to enable students to actualize the understanding inherent in Breema, and to express that understanding in his classes at the Breema Center. The dynamic atmosphere and aliveness of the Breema Center is a result of the efforts of the many students who have shown deep interest in and gratitude for Breema as a method of bodywork and a practical philosophy of living.

Breema Doesn't Need a Mystique

Malichek never gave a start-to-finish chronological picture of his life in Breema because he considered it to be tangential to his subject, and therefore, of no importance. His emphasis was always on bringing the principles and practice of Breema to life. His answers to questions that stemmed from mere curiosity were always brief. "Don't create more images for people," he told me. "Everyone has enough imaginary images that they try to fulfill. Breema doesn't need a mystique. To do Breema, you need to be ordinary. The magic of anything is the fact it exists. If you're looking for magic, you'll find it in the knowledge that you exist. Breema is a Universal principle. It doesn't belong to anyone in particular. Everyone could become a Breema student, a Breema instructor, or a master of Breema. What is needed is sincerity, honesty, and simplicity."

When I am alive,
When I am alert,
When I am connected to the
commonsense and instinctive
wisdom of my body,
Whatever I do is Breema.

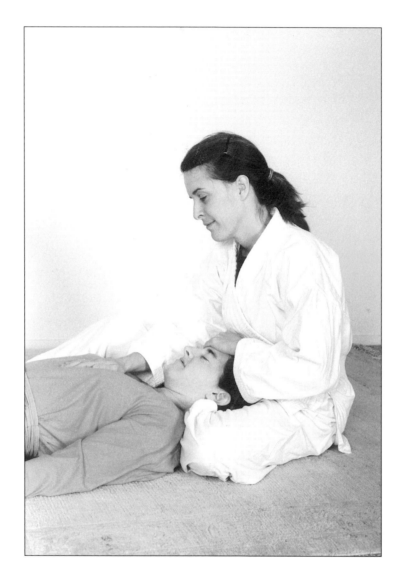

*Combinations of the level of Consciousness, energy, and matter
are all manifested Awareness.
We are "asleep" because we believe we exist
independently of the Unity of Existence.
To **wake up** means to know Existence exists
as one unified whole.*

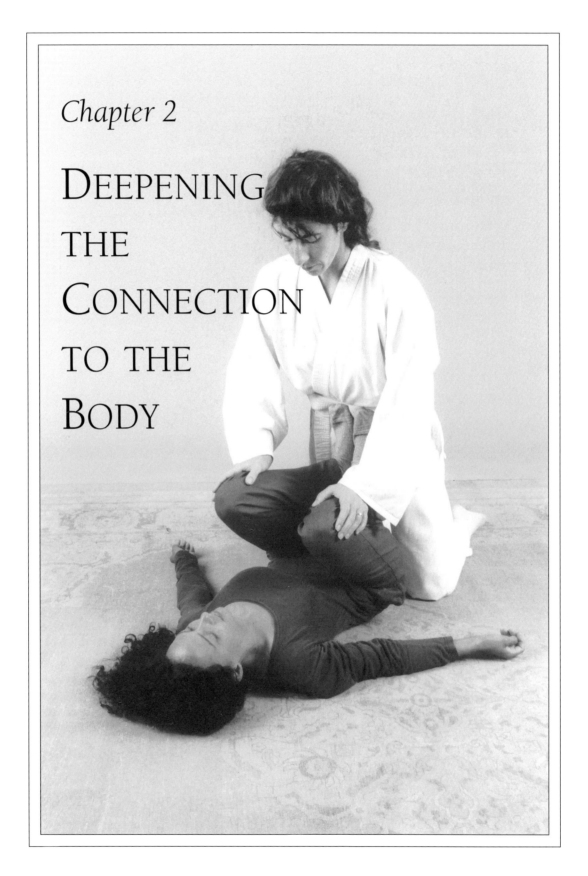

Chapter 2

DEEPENING THE CONNECTION TO THE BODY

A friend of mine returned from a long trip.

"How are things?" I asked him.

"Everything's a mess!" he told me. "My home is wrecked. The roof leaks, the foundation is cracked, I even found some termite damage."

"How long have you been away?" I asked.

"Almost a year," he said.

"Almost a year, and your house is falling apart? How old are you?" I asked.

"Thirty."

*"You've been on vacation from your body for thirty years. What do you think is happening **there**?"*

DEEPENING THE CONNECTION TO THE BODY

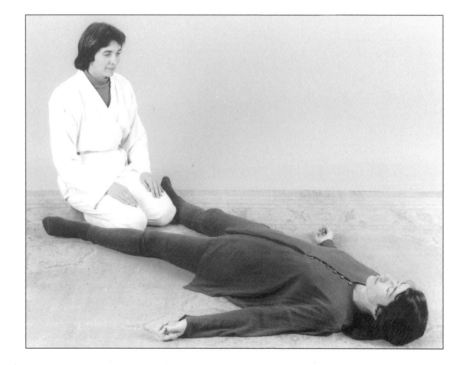

Connection to the body means connection to the *knowledge* that "there is a body." When I do Breema, I want to *know* that my body has weight, that my body is breathing. When I have this knowledge, I have something new. The part that can know *body breathes* has to be developed. The mind can *register* the body's weight and breathing. But the part that *knows* it is created by the desire of the mind, the desire of the feelings, and the desire of the body, unified and working together.

Deepening one's connection to the body is a part of deepening one's connection to Existence. The aim of Breema is unity, and in this *inclusive* Existence, body, mind, feelings, essence, Being, and Consciousness all are connected and receive their light from Awareness. When we give a non-judgmental treatment, we're taking a step towards unifying all levels of Existence. To do so, we need our Consciousness to function free of thoughts and feelings, and be receptive to the presence of Awareness. Breema is a method that starts with the most basic level, yet it aims for *Awakening*. To be *awake* means to be in the *moment*.

Meet Breema simply, un-philosophically, joyfully, and receptively. Your understanding will deepen with time.

Body Breathing, Body Comfortable

Practicing Breema, we work with our normal breathing rhythm. This rhythm, just as it is, is usually the most beneficial one for our body. If we could change that with our mind, that change would be unrelated to our physical need, because we don't understand our physical need sufficiently to properly change our rhythm. So, it's better not to try to change it. Just let it be.

However, in the course of giving or receiving a treatment, your body may pick up a message, effortlessly, and a change may take place in your breathing. That is safe, because your emphasis remains the comfort of the body. Don't interfere with your body's rhythm. Your breathing is based on the wisdom and intelligence of your body.

The intelligence of your body is sufficient to keep it going for seventy years or so. The rhythm of your breathing constantly changes in response to many factors. Every thought, every memory provokes a change in rhythm. Your instinctive intelligence uses your breathing to buffer the effect of your psychological state on your body.

When you do Breema, it's important to make your body comfortable. It doesn't matter how many times you need to change your position to be comfortable — do so! There is no outer aim to take priority over being comfortable in your postures and movements. By constantly "coming back" to make sure your body is comfortable and that you are registering your own weight and breath, you're supporting yourself to have *connection to the body,* and to give a non-judgmental treatment.

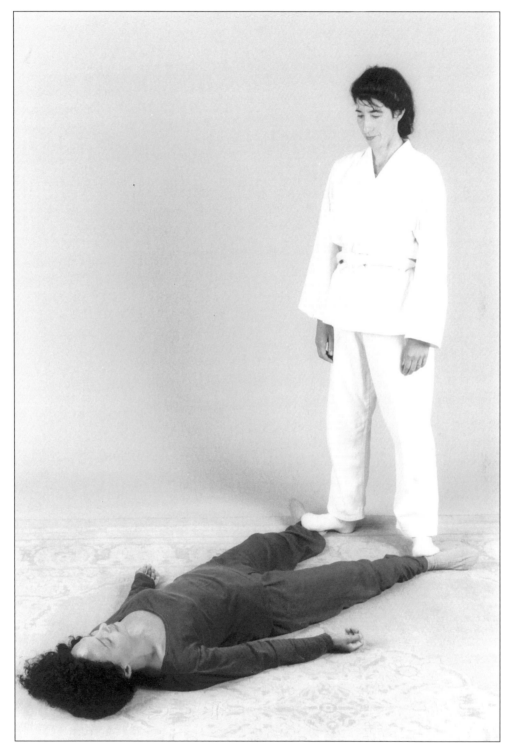

Many Breema treatments begin with the feet placed on the heels.

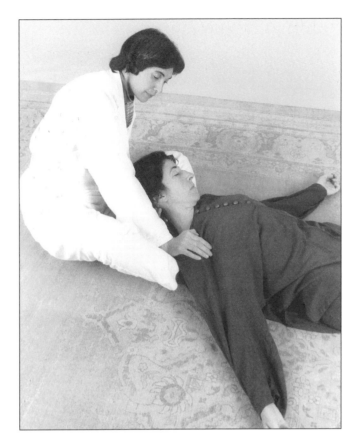

The Recipient Is *Your* Opportunity

Let the *body* work, free of concern about what others may think or feel about your treatment.

Bring your attention to register that your body has weight and breathes. Now your attention is not on others. Correct use of your attention is just the beginning. It's the "starter," not the engine. Practicing Breema, you receive energy not just from the mind, but also from the levels of Consciousness and Awareness.

By applying this principle, you can connect the mind, feelings, and body, which usually work without any connection to each other. The emphasis is always on your own growth, not the person you are working on. The recipient is *your* opportunity to benefit by the activity of giving a treatment. That experience is your teacher, and you, its student. That's why we end every treatment by bowing to the recipient. When you're doing Breema just for yourself, the highest gift becomes available to the recipient, too — the gift of being accepted in unity.

Let the Body Move Naturally

Let your body move naturally. Your mind doesn't know how to move your body. When you let your mind tell the body what to do, all your postures and movements are stiff. You become uncomfortable and filled with tension. Your feelings don't know how to move your body either. They make your movements exaggerated. They use up too much energy. They imitate others blindly.

Your body knows how to sit. It knows how to walk and move. It learns how to give a treatment. All of Breema's movements and postures are natural and instinctive for your body. All you need is a little practice, with the mind and emotions supporting. Let the mind register weight, breath, and movement. Let the feelings support the body's activities with the calm enthusiasm of their natural presence.

This way, your body moves naturally, and your mind adds a quality of interest and purposefulness to that movement. Your feelings add presence and the substance of joy to your movement. Bringing these three to work together as partners is what the treatment is all about.

*Existence is one
Timeless Moment —
this moment.*

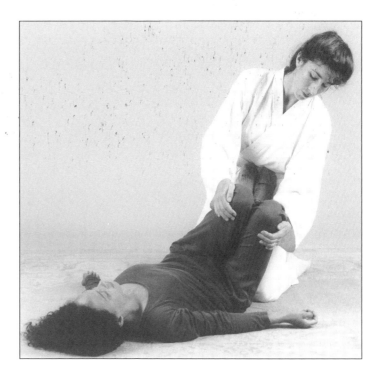

Use Your Whole Body

At the beginning of many treatments, you bring your partner's foot up onto your leg. According to the principle of *using your whole body,* you are not allowed to "lift," because as soon as you lift, you create an energy blockage at your shoulder, since you're using force. By using force, the body is divided. Your arm is separated from the energy in the rest of your body by the tension in your shoulder. And the principle says, "whatever you do, do it with all of your body."

What you can do is to connect with your body and lean forward and then lean back. In the process of this leaning forward and backward, your partner's foot comes up onto your leg without effort.

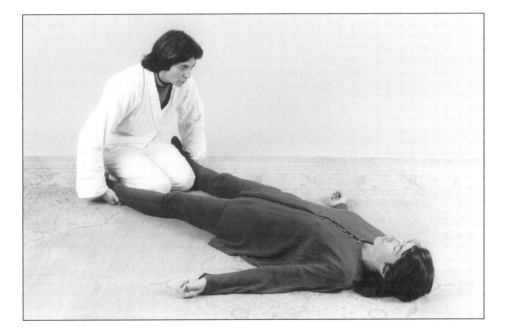

Staying Connected with Your Partner

It is important to maintain as much physical connection as is comfortable with your partner when practicing, because the treatment deposits a new "food" in the body.

While you're eating, it's best to let your body relax, and not be too active. Your digestive organs need energy and time to digest the food you've eaten. The process of "digesting" the treatment is the same. In order for the body to assimilate that new food, you have to give it extra support in the form of continued contact. This allows your partner to absorb the effects of the treatment much more fully, because they become more open and receptive. It allows the treatment to penetrate to a deeper level.

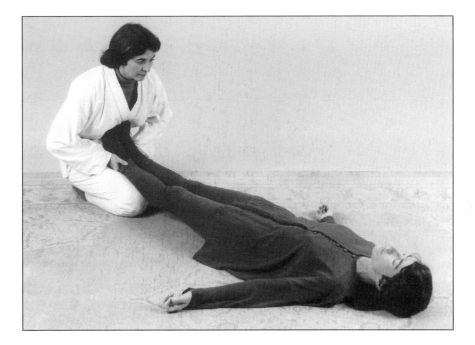

*The Field of Existence is **inclusive**, and is beyond words and concepts.*
It cannot be conceptualized by the mind,
and as soon as words are used to describe it,
they are approximate.

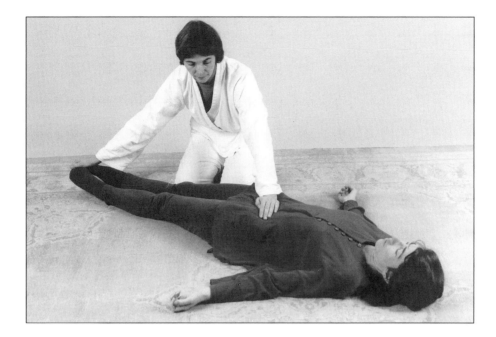

Holding for Three Breaths

One characteristic of life energy is that it has an attractive force. It attracts more life to itself. When we hold during a treatment, we allow the body's natural compassion to manifest because our touch does not need to be guided by our mind. That's how a mother holds her baby — naturally, without thinking of how to hold. By allowing our body's natural compassion to manifest without interference, our mind and our feelings can also learn to have this quality. Usually, the energy fields of the two bodies are acquainted after holding for three breaths at the beginning of a sequence.

When we hold, there is no pause, no discontinuity in the treatment. Our holding is active and at the same time, receptive. The body is an energy system, and like everything in the Universe, it has constant motion and is interconnected with everything else. Every stone, every grain of sand is in motion. There is nothing that is not alive.

Leaning

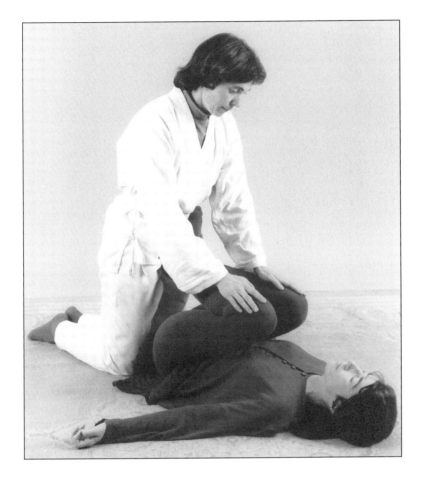

When you lean into any part of the recipient's body, for instance, while leaning the legs towards the recipient's abdomen, your relaxed attention should be on your own body. As you lean in, all the principles are expressed: your body is comfortable, your whole body is participating in the lean, and the movement is complete within each second. Your weight totally supports the recipient's body. Effortlessly, without losing your connection to your own body, your *body* naturally senses any "correction" the recipient's body needs, and without doing anything extra, their pelvis and vertebrae realign themselves naturally as your weight sinks in. No diagnostic process is necessary. Nor do you need to visualize or imagine anything. Your mind functions supportively by registering, without tension, your own body's weight and breathing.

Treatments often combine stretching and leaning. Leaning in helps the body to accept greater stretches. Stretching opens the body so it can receive deeper leans.

Lean with the Natural Weight of the Body

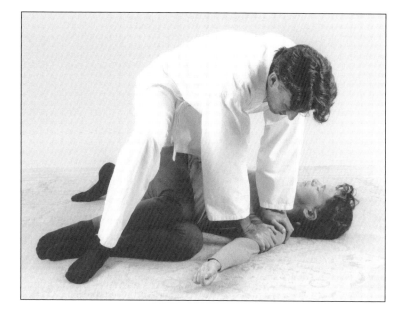

When you lean into the recipient's body, communication is established. The amount of weight the recipient's body "asks for" may vary from one treatment to the next, and from day to day. When your body "gets it," there's no uncertainty. When you lean in, using the relaxed, natural weight of the body, your instinctive part determines how much is enough. While you're learning, the rule of thumb is: if it's uncomfortable, it's not right. If the recipient tenses slightly, that's natural. If they tense more than that, *you're* not completely comfortable. When you're connected to your body, you can lean in with a lot of weight. When you're tense or judgmental, even a little weight is unacceptable.

Leaning has three components — a gradual lean, a hold, and a gradual release. Doing lean-hold-release is like offering the recipient a meal. The lean is like serving the food. The more slowly you lean in, the better, so that trust can be established. The hold is like eating the meal. The slow release allows the meal to be digested. You can feel how deep to go. If the recipient can't take much weight, their body will communicate that to your body. As the recipient becomes more open, their body may accept more of your body weight. But remember that more weight and deeper leaning doesn't make a better treatment. Your presence and participation is what makes the treatment more penetrating. Even the lightest touch, when it has the qualities of firmness and gentleness, enables the recipient to extract exactly what they need from the treatment to come to a state of balance.

Your rhythm must be smooth, although you can vary the tempo. Avoid hesitation, because your uncertainty is transmitted to the recipient, who then remains guarded. When the recipient is less receptive, and you feel some resistance to the treatment, try slowing down your movement. Move more gradually. Lean in a little less. At the same time, give more support to their body.

Leaning Isn't Doing, It's Participating

Even when we say the word "push" or "pull," we tense up — that's the effect of these words!

Whenever we *do* anything, our mind is the boss. Pushing and pulling are *doing*. Leaning isn't doing, it's *participating*. When we participate in life, we benefit.

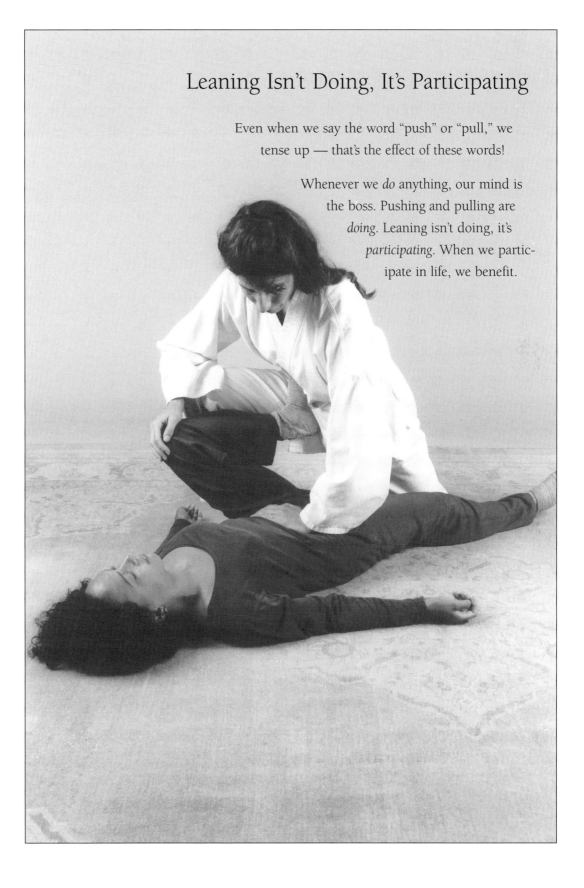

Brushing

Many Breema treatments include brushing. Brushing communicates completion and security to the body, and allows the parts of the treatment that preceded it to penetrate and affect the body more deeply.

Most brushes are done either three or seven times. Counting helps your mind stay involved.

We don't brush "with the arm," because brushing with the arm alone divides the body, blocks the energy at the shoulder, and as a result, blocks the flow of energy between the arm and the rest of the body.

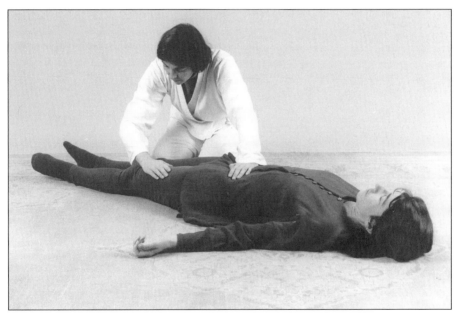

Brushing from the abdomen down the left leg.

You simply let your hand rest on the body, then your whole body leans back. Your *body* does the brushing, and your hand is an extension of your body. Since your hand doesn't *do* anything, there is no reason for it to be tense. Your hand is so relaxed, it molds to the contours of the part it's brushing, and it makes full contact, constantly. Your whole body participates when you brush.

You're really learning that your body is one unit. The mind divides your body for you — this is your right hand, your little finger, your thumb nail. Even when we work with one part, we express it a little differently. We say "body's hand" or "body's eyes." The emphasis always remains with the fact of the body as one unit.

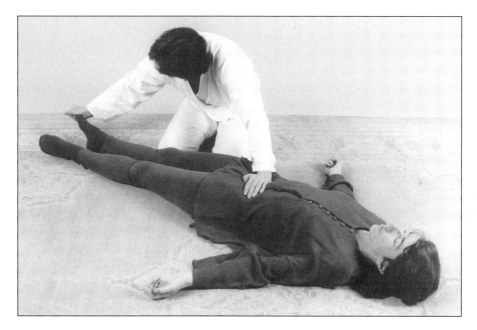

Brushing from the abdomen down the right leg.

Let Your Body Do the Treatment

Practicing Breema, you learn to shift the emphasis to yourself. All our lives we haven't included ourselves in the impressions we receive of life. Now slowly you shift your emphasis, and include yourself.

The mind doesn't know how to do Breema. The feelings don't know how to do Breema. But when you stay with the experience of your own body, and register your own breathing, weight, and level of comfort, your body knows how to do Breema.

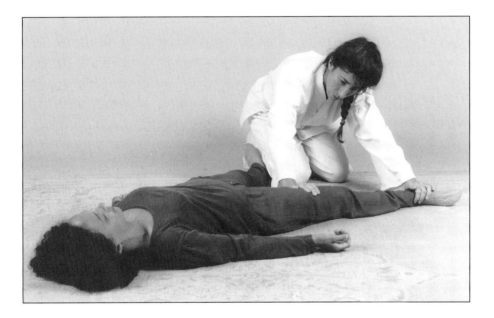

Our body is one element of the organic life on the planet Earth.
The purpose of our body cannot be separate from the purpose of organic life on Earth,
just as one cell in the tip of our finger can't have a purpose
different from the purpose of our body as a whole.

Let your *body* do the treatment.

The body is more than atoms and molecules, just as your shoes are more than leather and rubber. The intelligence of the shoemaker and the design and purpose of the shoes are also part of the shoes. In the same way, Consciousness and Awareness are part of the body.

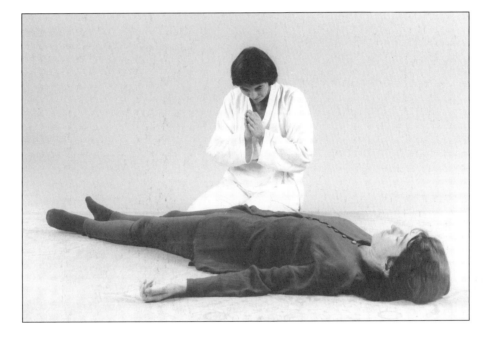

Every treatment ends by bowing to the recipient as an expression of gratitude
for the opportunity afforded the practitioner to balance their own energy,
experience their own body, and unify their own mind, feelings, and body.

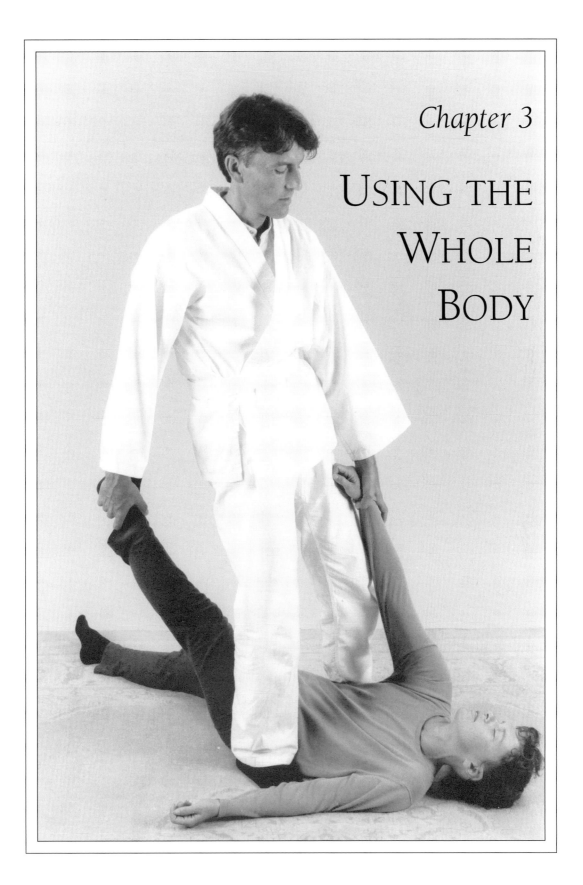

Chapter 3

USING THE
WHOLE
BODY

Whatever you do,
do it with all of you.

USING THE
WHOLE BODY

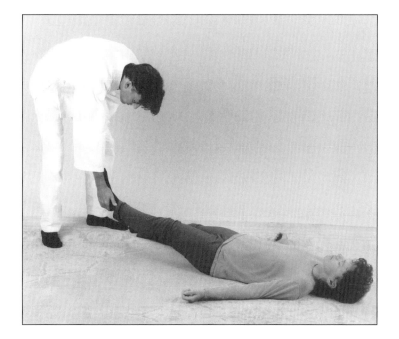

In order for me to do Breema, everything I do has to involve all of me. That means full participation. Life energy flows through the body as a *whole*, not through one part. If I don't understand that the body is *one unit*, I think one hand is brushing, and my other hand is holding the abdomen. This separation is exactly what Breema bypasses. Because it is not guided by my thinking process, it lets my mind simply register. It registers the body having weight and breathing. This is exactly what I need in order to harmonize my mind, body, and feelings. This simple practice of registering the body's weight and breathing is the foundation of Breema. From the very beginning, we work with this registration, so it becomes an integral part of any treatment we do.

If you perform a movement using only your arm, for example, it's not Breema. Your arm is being used as a mechanical tool. But when your arm functions as a part of your whole body, then it's no longer just your arm doing the treatment. Your energy is flowing, and your arm becomes a *living* tool.

No force is necessary. No strain or extra muscular work is required. In fact, you experience no "extra," because your movement lets the recipient's body function as an integral part of *your* body. Whatever you do, you do with all of you.

You can call this an elbow. You can call this a knee. But really, there's just one body. If you work with this principle, you'll eventually understand that it's the key to creating a nurturing atmosphere.

When we practice a treatment, we're touching with our hand. We may call this a hand, but there's really no separation. There is just one body. The hand never works separately from the whole body. Unless your whole body is relaxed when you touch the recipient, your hand won't mold itself to the exact contours of the body it's touching. The communication between the two bodies and the two energy fields is not total. Full contact allows you to both give and receive total support.

Completion in Movement

Any movement you make during a treatment needs to reach completion. That means you continue the movement until you experience it as complete, full, satisfying. If you're leaning, lean until your weight has settled in, and it feels as though every cell of your body has "arrived" and become a part of your new momentary posture. Once you experience completion, move on. Every movement of the treatment is experienced as a complete moment by itself. You never hurry, yet never pause.

*The truth of Existence can only be tasted in **unconditioned** Consciousness.*

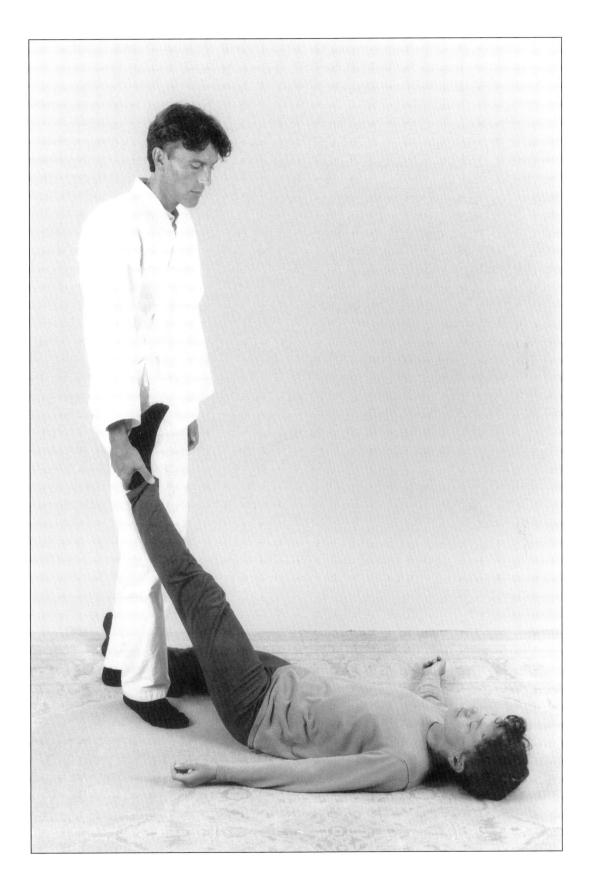

The Breema Principles

I tell everyone who studies with me: Look for one thing, and don't cheat yourself — try to get the principles. A principle is something that can be applied in everything you do. You could apply it when you drink a glass of water, when you shake hands with someone, when you smile or talk, in fact, anytime. These principles are something you can use. Everything else will eventually become mechanical for you, and you won't benefit from it. If you don't make Breema yours, it will just be something you learned mechanically, by imitating what somebody else did. After awhile it will lose its aliveness for you, and you'll lose your interest in it. But if you learn the principles, you can use what you learn in many different ways, and Breema will always remain alive for you.

Whatever I do, my aim is to actually know that I am doing it. This means that when I touch someone's body, the purpose is for me to actually *experience* what I am doing. The mind can't experience what I'm doing. The feelings can't experience what I'm doing. Even the body can't have the full experience of touching. But when mind, body, and feelings work together *simultaneously,* I can experience whatever I am doing. If just my mind says my body is touching (or sitting, or walking), I am settling for a definition and concept of my activity. I still don't *experience* my activity. If only my feelings say I am touching, it's incomplete. If only my body says so, it's incomplete. None of these three have any real authority by themselves. But when my mind, feelings, and body are unified in my activity, the *experience* of touching also becomes part of the activity. The experience is what makes that activity tangible.

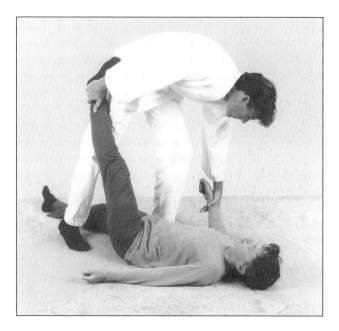

After a while,
you will enjoy Breema
so much.

Rhythm is there.
Momentum is created.
Your body constantly enjoys it.
You wish to keep
going with it.
Your whole body is active
as one unit.
In every movement
you have a taste of
being supported by Existence.

Understanding the Breema Principles

The principles of Breema can be understood on many levels. Superficially, you can relate them to concepts you've already heard. In that case, the principles will remain theoretical.

Another level is reached by actually looking to see if the principles make sense in terms of your own life experience. The principles can affect you more deeply still if you let yourself be open and receptive to them, reading the words and terms used as though hearing them for the first time. Even more useful is to practice applying them. The principles take on an entirely new meaning when they are alive for you in the moment.

It's just like describing a pomegranate. Someone who has never seen one gets a certain idea of what you mean. Someone who has seen a pomegranate understands you more closely. Someone who has eaten one has a more precise idea of what you're talking about. But, someone who is eating one while you're talking knows exactly what you mean. Their understanding of the word is alive.

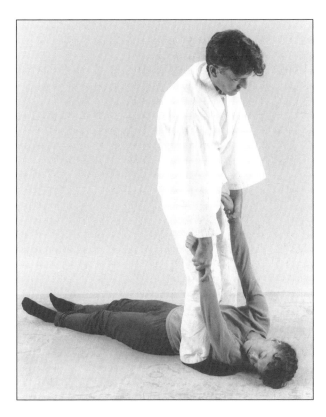

Whole Body Participates

We say "use your whole body." Yet the whole body cannot be separate from the whole person. When all four levels of Existence (Awareness, Consciousness, energy, and matter) are present, the word "whole" is correctly used.

Your mind and feelings can become receptive and available while your body is active. When this is the case, Consciousness and Awareness can also participate as presence and watchfulness. Watchfulness doesn't mean something is watching something else. Watchfulness means Awareness is shining through. One *is* and manifests as Existence. In this way, any simple activity of the body becomes a sacred dance that gives the taste of "I exist."

Natural Rhythm of the Body

Everything our life depends on is rhythmic — the cycle of day and night, the cycle of the moon, our heartbeat, our breathing. Many of our cells communicate with each other through rhythm. All of our organs have a rhythm, which is the general rhythm of the body. Our connection to the Earth is re-established via rhythm.

When we find our natural rhythm doing Breema, and work with it, we are energized and refreshed, and life is enjoyable. Using the momentum and rhythm natural to our movement, our own energy is conserved and revitalized.

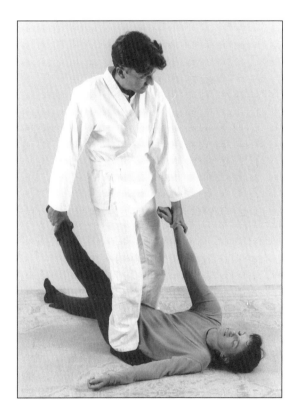

From the moment of our conception, our body has a rhythm.
We begin life with this rhythm, which is in harmony with the Earth and the rest of the Universe,
but as we grow up, we receive an imbalanced education that overemphasizes the mind.
Our mind learns to dominate us, causing illness and unhappiness.
When we rediscover our natural rhythm, we take a step towards living a balanced life.

Mutual Support — Mutual Benefit

Whenever you can increase the support you're giving to the recipient, do so. You can never give too much support. Support is created by having more contact, but most especially, by being more present.

The more you apply the principles while practicing a treatment, the more your body, mind, and feelings receive exactly what they need from the treatment in order to become balanced and vital. And the amazing thing is that as you're doing the treatment "for yourself," the recipient also receives just what they need from the treatment.

As you become more experienced, your body's instinctive wisdom chooses which treatment sequences to practice at a particular time. Because it's receptive to the energy field created by both you and the recipient together, your body's instinctive wisdom chooses the treatments that will give both of you the greatest benefit.

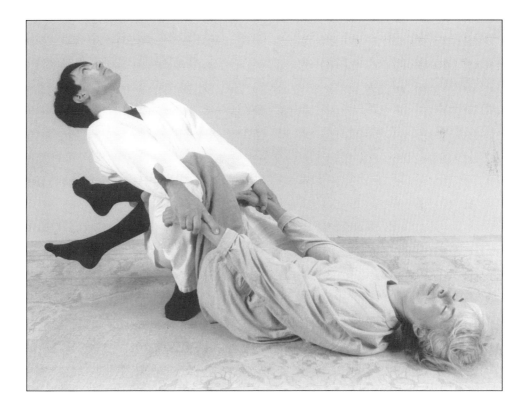

The principle of *mutual support,* like every Breema principle, also applies when you're not practicing Breema bodywork, but are in the current of daily affairs.

Say, for example, a friend comes to visit you. While you are greeting her, you know your body has weight and breathes. Your handshake is firm and gentle, and invites your friend to be balanced with you.

The principle of *mutual support — mutual benefit* doesn't end with the physical aspect of the treatment. It can extend into every moment of our lives.

If your body is not enjoying it, you're not doing Breema, because there is no movement in Breema which is not an expression of joy.

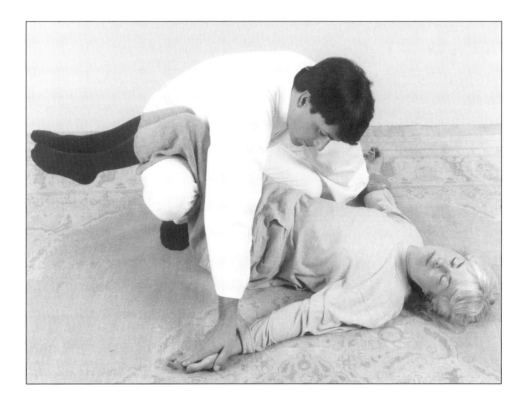

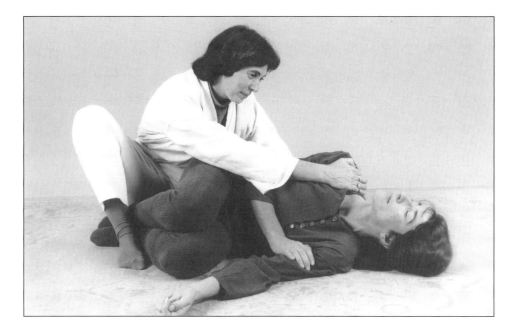

When we say "use your whole body," we're not only referring to the physical body. It means doing something with the participation of your permanent aspect. Whole means that which takes place at the presence of the Field of Existence. To really use your whole body, you can't remain separate from Existence, because whole means the whole of Existence.

An atmosphere of acceptance is a natural expression of the knowledge that, in truth, *only the Field of Existence exists.* We cannot have acceptance of something we view as incomplete or separate. This is why Breema is non-diagnostic. It constantly refers both practitioner and recipient to the whole — working with the whole, moving with it, talking with it, touching with it. All of this means that you know you exist. And this "you," although tangible in Consciousness without thought, cannot be pointed to, or defined, or seen. This "you" exists as part of Existence as a whole.

When the definite Knowledge that "I exist" is present,
the mind, feelings, and body simultaneously receive an impression of it,
and yet that knowledge is itself independent of the mind, feelings, and body.
The knowledge that "I exist" is tangible, yet inseparable from the whole.

Moving with Full Participation

Use your whole body in every movement, in everything you do. Chew food with your whole body. Move your hand with your whole body. By practicing, you learn what that means. When, during a treatment, you bring the recipient's legs up onto your lap, your aim is to do it as though all the cells in your body, even the cells at the tips of your toes, are participating.

When your aim is to use your whole body in any activity, even the parts of your body that don't have much to do with the physical movement become supportive. With practice, this instinctive way of moving becomes natural to you, and your total energy participates in your every movement. When mind, feelings, and body work together, your movements, whether part of a treatment or not, have a balancing quality. Just watching someone who moves with full participation is nurturing.

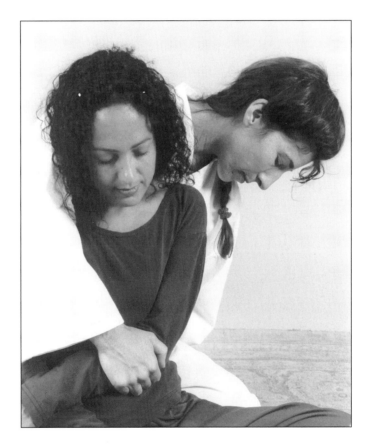

Body Relaxed

Good practitioners emanate relaxation — through their eyes, breathing, facial expressions, posture, tone of voice, gestures, and movements. The way they listen, shake hands, touch, and smile is relaxed. The practitioner's attitude is that relaxation is the gift of harmony with one's surroundings, and this gift is given whenever we are available to receive it. This way, the practitioner finds a compassionate posture towards life.

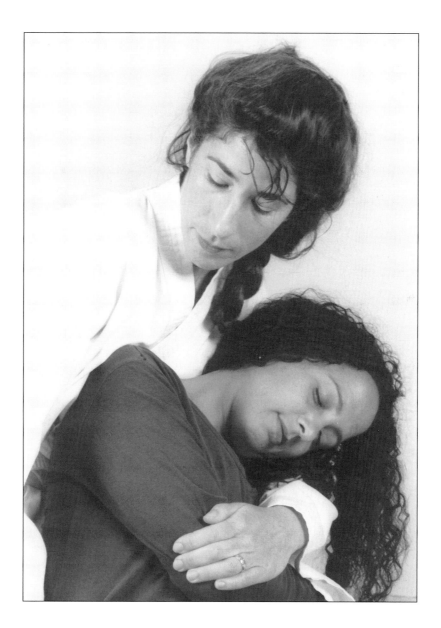

Remember — Stay Comfortable

Don't hesitate to move your partner's body or your own body around to get comfortable.

When your emphasis is on making your body comfortable, your concerns about making your partner feel good disappear, and with them, judgment disappears. In its place there is a quality of acceptance that allows your partner to be open to receive that which they need at that moment. Their *Being* is nurtured.

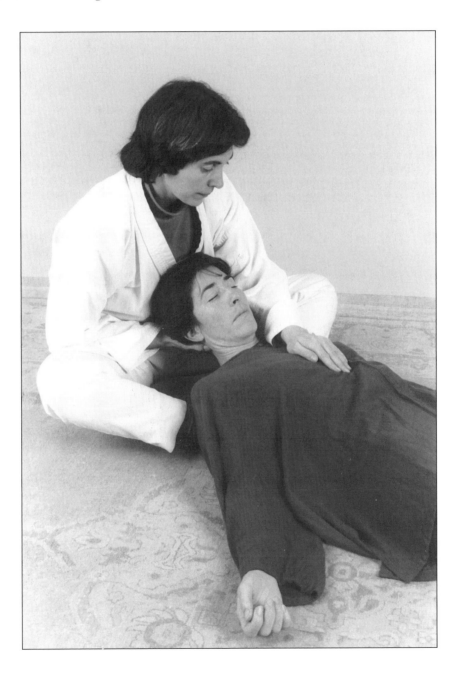

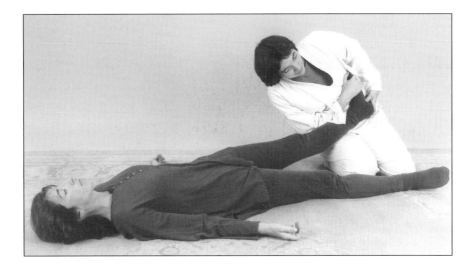

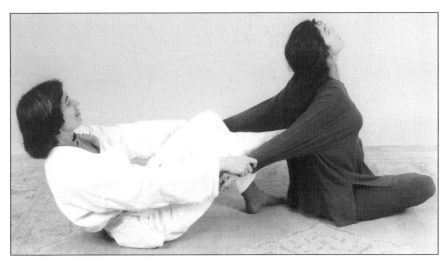

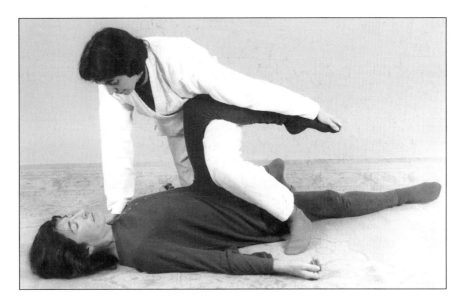

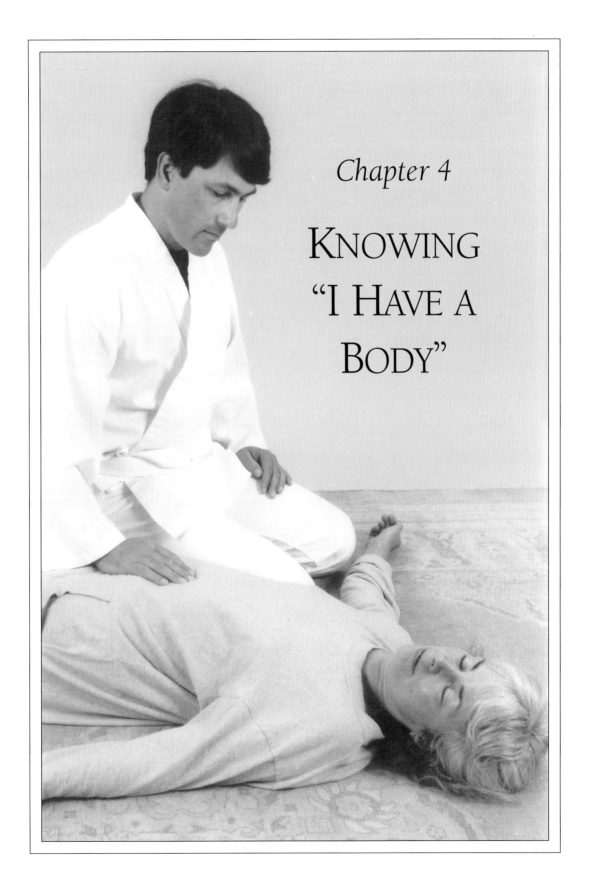

Chapter 4

KNOWING
"I HAVE A
BODY"

When my mind, feelings, and body
function together as one unit,
I have my own center of gravity.

KNOWING
"I HAVE A BODY"

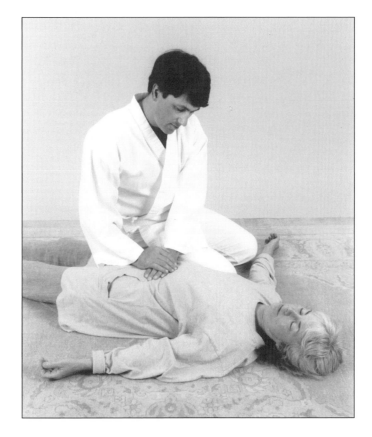

The definite *knowing* that "I have a body" is not dependent on tension, physical sensation, or physical location. At first, these may be part of our experience. As our experience increases, it becomes freer and freer, until only the knowledge of "there is a body" remains. This knowing doesn't have a sense of separation, a line separating "me" from that which is "outside of me." In fact, we are more connected to our surroundings. The knowledge of "I have a body" is the beginning of the knowledge that Existence exists.

When we have the definite taste of "I have a body" or "there is a body," there is no longer any need to emphasize one part of the body over any other part. That "taste" is a *knowledge* which is equally the property of every cell of the body. Every cell of the body is working together, and the *knowledge* of this is your vital center, your center of gravity. When you are connected to this knowledge, the energy you use to do a treatment is continually replenished. This is the self-vitalizing aspect of Breema.

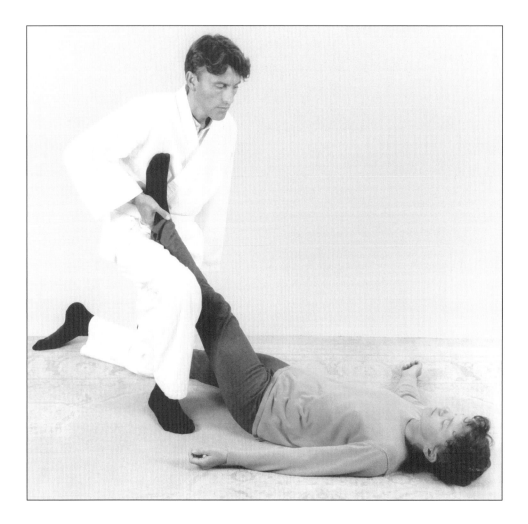

Only when the knowledge of "there is a body" is present in us, is it possible to have new, uncrystallized postures, movements, facial expressions, tones of voice, and gestures. These uncrystallized physical manifestations act to decrystallize our mind and "feelings," so we can have new thoughts and proper feelings. When body, mind, and feelings all are experienced, we have a sense of *presence*. The mind is receptive and clear. The feelings are centered and free. The body has original, *organic* sensations, and flexibility. These qualities should not be searched for or imagined. When they become present, they let us know. That knowing eventually becomes *Being-knowledge.* This harmonizing knowledge is the threshold that leads to freedom from what we think we are, and moves us towards what we actually are, towards the knowledge of "I exist." Although "I exist" has a personal taste, it excludes nothing and is a part of Existence as a whole. It is the beginning of the profound Understanding of the Unity of all things that all religions and Objective Science have as their aim.

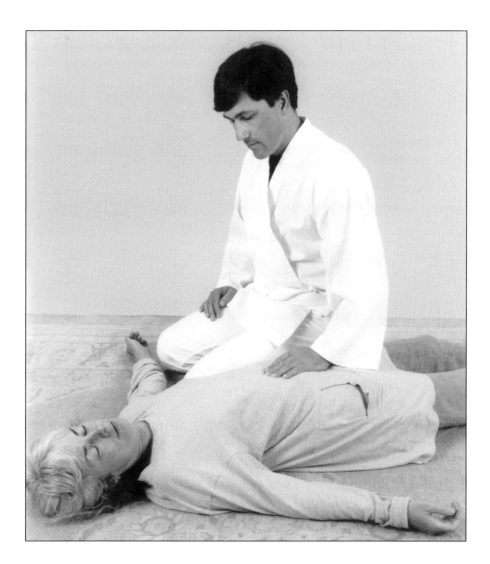

It is important to rely on your own experience, with full acceptance, no matter how small your experience is. Receive it as a precious gift given by Existence to help you become a unified presence, belonging to the whole. Let your small experiences remain *personal* treasures, gifts given to you. It isn't really necessary to talk about these experiences, because no matter how small they are, they announce themselves through their own emanation and radiation. Just enjoy being ordinary, and be grateful you're on the right track.

The energy gained from these small moments can be used in your ordinary daily life to accomplish some of the things you've wished to do, things which have been put off through inertia and the tendency to postpone "for later." In due time, these small accomplishments make us capable of bigger accomplishments, like losing our false sense of specialness and importance, and gaining an accurate posture of respect for oneself as a *Being-participant* on the Earth. The person who sees that his mind, and feelings, and body (which are *form*) are at any moment, subject to disappear completely, as is everything his eyes come to rest on, can have true respect for his existence on the Earth, and for Existence as a whole.

Connection to the Knowledge of "There Is a Body"

Once you register the fact "there is a body," you will see that most of the time you are not connected to this knowledge. When you see that, you have to be grateful, because that knowledge is your *aim*. Seeing you don't have it means you can take the next step. Maybe that step is to experience the weight of your body, or to know you are breathing. At any given moment, your aim is something you can do, not something impossible. That way, you can always take a step in the right direction.

When we say Earth, we're not talking philosophically about the planet. We're talking about *our* Earth — our own body. When we're connected to the knowledge of "there is a body," we are on the Earth.

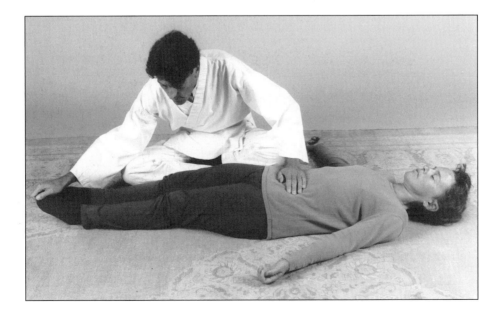

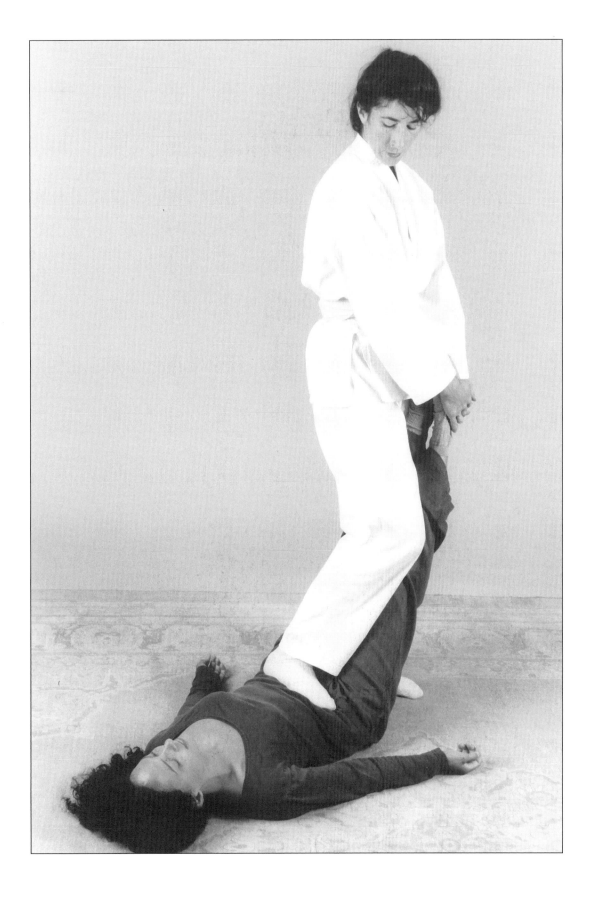

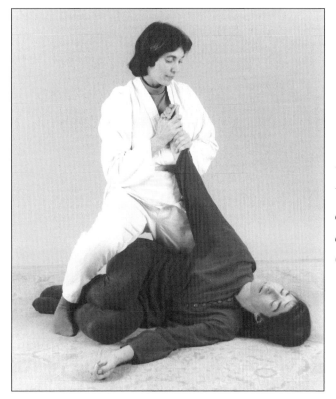

The emphasis is not on "fixing" others.
You just manifest
according to your Being,
doing what feels right for you.
Others are helped by it.

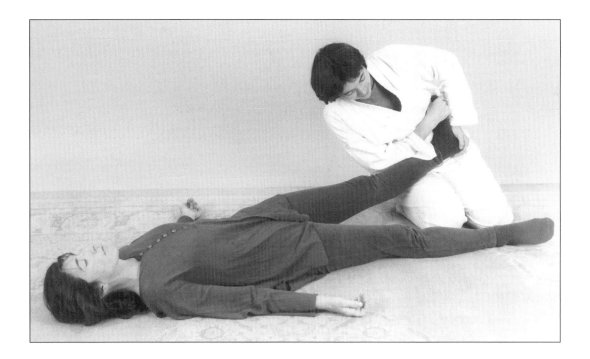

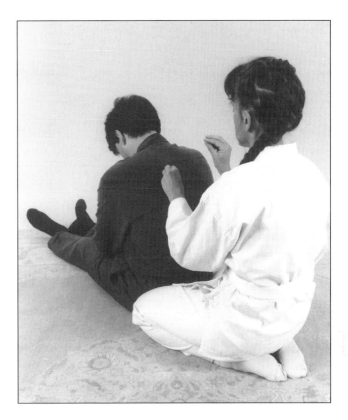

The Sun, with his very essence,
wishes to shine.
He doesn't say, "I am helping you."
But you are welcome to use his light
and heat.

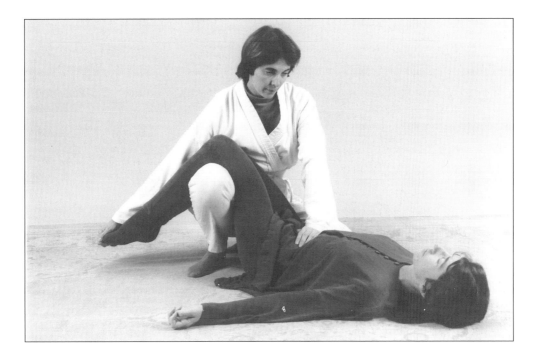

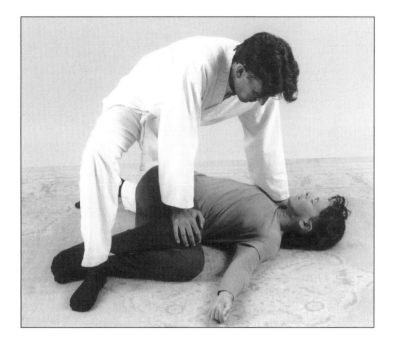

The Interest of the Mind

Our mind has been "educated" to record, retrieve, compare, and classify information. But when we repeat what we've heard or read, our words are hollow, because we don't really *know* what we're talking about! We don't experience an inner satisfaction when we mechanically present our mind's accumulated information as something we actually know, because that information hasn't become part of our *Being*.

When the mind becomes interested in registering the activity of our own body, we have more energy, because instead of separating itself from our body, the mind starts to *participate* in our body's activity. As we continue to register our body's manifestations with interest, our feelings start to participate too, and we experience a new quality of aliveness.

When an *inner authority* is created through the unification of our body, mind, and feelings, and through our desire for self-understanding, an impression of Existence is simultaneously received in all three. In fact, this *I* exists in the absence of thoughts and feelings. At the presence of that authority, we are connected to Existence. We remain ordinary, but life "tastes" different — the taste of I-AMness is in it.

"Do you know what freedom is?" Malichek once asked me. "I thought I did," I said, "until you asked." "*Everything* in life is like that," he said. "Do you know you are standing here? At first, we assume we know about everything. But when that authority which *knows* you have a body exists, you have freedom from conceptual existence."

Our mind, by itself, cannot be a source of understanding.
Understanding is the union of sound knowledge and Being.

The Aim of Breema

Breema can relax us, but that's not its principal aim. Breema decrystallizes the body, mind, and feelings. As the body is decrystallized, it becomes capable of having new movements and postures. Its relationship to the life force changes.

As the feelings are decrystallized, they no longer try to use the body as a vehicle for self-expression.

As the mind is decrystallized, mind, feelings, and body can have a new relationship and function cooperatively.

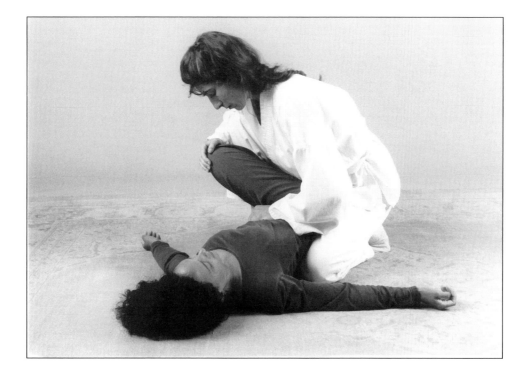

Breema's principles don't say your mind or feelings have to be a certain way.
Breema is simply a way of freeing energy for productive work.
Whatever you wish to do, you need energy to do it.
Associative mind, reactive feelings, and tense body waste energy.
Working with the principles creates receptive mind, supportive feelings, and relaxed body.
The energy which is usually consumed by the conflict between mind and feelings,
and by physical tension, becomes available.

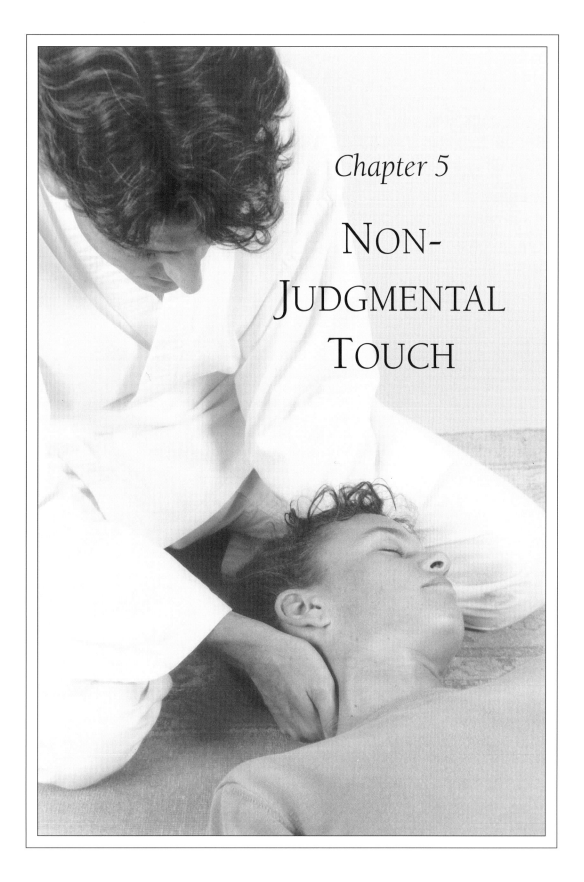

Chapter 5

NON-
JUDGMENTAL
TOUCH

The root of vitality is in the Awareness of Existence.

NON-JUDGMENTAL
TOUCH

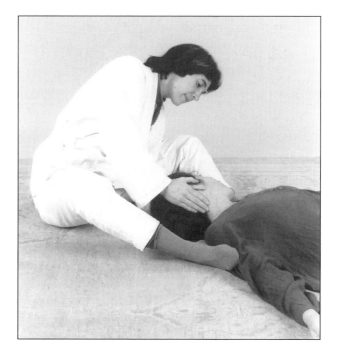

There is *one* body. You are not separate from the recipient. This unity is the foundation of Breema. The key is to see that we are not this body, not this mind, not these feelings. These three aspects are *events* of life. Our Awareness and Consciousness are not events — they are the core substance of our Existence. When I have a taste of "I exist," judgment disappears. When we believe we are our mind, feelings, and body, we are identified, and that which we observe, we justify, rather than accept. Breema begins with registering the fact that our body has weight and the fact that our body breathes, without feelings of like and dislike, and without taking the information from the registering part of the mind to the automatic flow of associations. In association, our energy and attention are drawn to the past or future.

The aim is acceptance of our own condition, and from there, acceptance of the condition of the recipient. This creates an atmosphere of acceptance in which the recipient has a chance to accept their own body. They simply let go of the "extra."

Ultimately, things are the only way they could be. Everything that happens is a necessary part of one whole. In the same way, there are many cells in our body. Every day, many are "born" and many "die." Each cell has a certain function, and does its job in the world of the body. Each lives a blameless life. Just so, we become one cell of this planet, and perform our function. When we take a bite of an apple, it is divided into many elements, life energy is extracted from it, and many aspects of our life are nurtured. A piece of wood on the ground eventually becomes soil. Everything is part of one harmony.

When we don't recognize this harmony, nothing makes sense. There is no understanding. We identify with the world of temporary appearance. To reach unity within ourselves, we have to unify our mind, feelings, and body. This is the first step towards raising our consciousness to a level that is free of judgment. When we have unified Consciousness, we see things *inclusively*, as they are. When we are free of judgment, we look, accept, and understand.

When we say "I exist," we're referring to a rare experience which
cannot be produced by the mind, the feelings, or by wishing alone.
*In order for the **I** to actually exist,*
total disidentification with our conceptual existence is necessary.
This is a completely new dimension,
which is not the domain of the person who is "asleep."

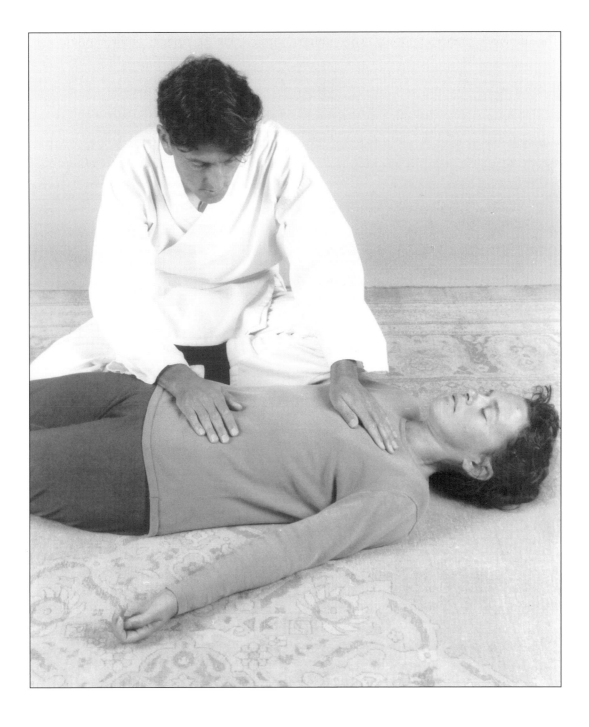

When I have a taste of "I exist," judgment disappears.

Non-Judgmental Treatment

In order for your partner to receive your treatment, you need to be non-judgmental while giving the treatment. If you touch someone as if they're sick, though their body may be imbalanced, you're touching only a small part of them. Every imbalance is temporary. You end up playing with the layers of muscle and skin, but you can't affect their *Being*. Everyone is really searching for acceptance and understanding. If you can touch non-judgmentally, it's possible to have an exchange on a much deeper level — the level of the inner wisdom which gives vitality at a moment's notice.

Your aim is to increase vitality, not to fight sickness. Your aim is to to give a non-judgmental treatment.

Our purpose for giving a treatment becomes to make our body flexible, to ask our mind to remain with the body's weight, breath, movement, and posture, and to have our feelings function supportively rather than reactively.

The treatment becomes an opportunity we use to bring ourselves into harmony and balance, and so creates a non-judgmental atmosphere that, by itself, gives the recipient more than the practitioner could give directly.

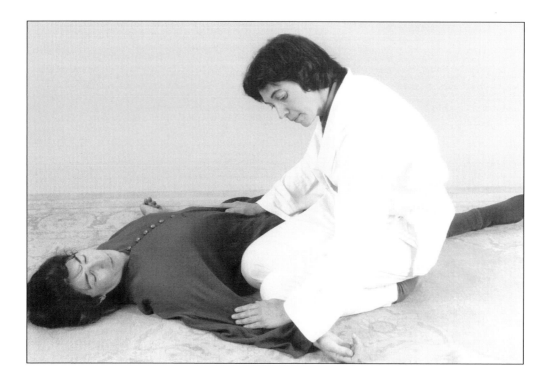

Tension

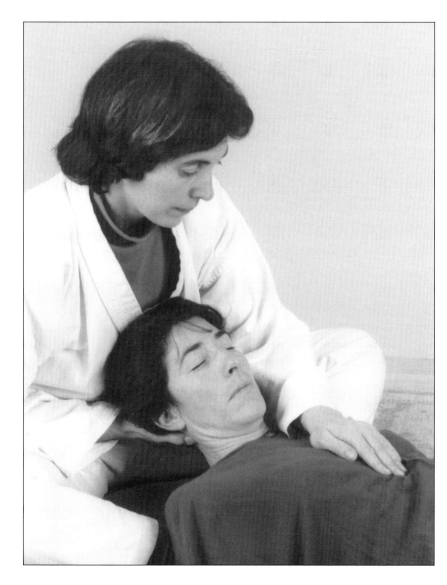

When we feel insecure or uncomfortable, we tense up. The more relaxed we are, the more strength we have. In the absense of tension, we are more vital. When we're tense, we fight gravity, instead of allowing ourselves to be supported by the ground we're standing on, the chair we're sitting on, or even the bed we're sleeping on.

There are five kinds of tension:

1. Tension which is created as a result of lack of interest in participating in where we are and what we're doing.

2. Tension which is created as a result of criticism of ourselves or others, or as a result of criticism of other people towards us.

3. Tension which is created as a result of not fulfilling that which we know we should do.

4. Tension which is created as a result of worry and fear.

5. Tension which is the result of the mismanagement of energy.

All people, animals, plants, and objects have an emanation which we receive and which affects us. We are affected by every experience life presents us. Our automatic, unconscious way of classifying everything, judging everything, and filtering everything through our associative thought chain prevents us from seeing things as they are, so that which we receive is not truth.

Tension is created by the conflict between the reality of things as they are, and our preconceptions and associations.

We think that we know how to release our tension by relaxing the tense part. But what we are actually doing is shunting tension to another area. Tension is a symptom, just as a headache is. Relaxing does not get to the root of the cause.

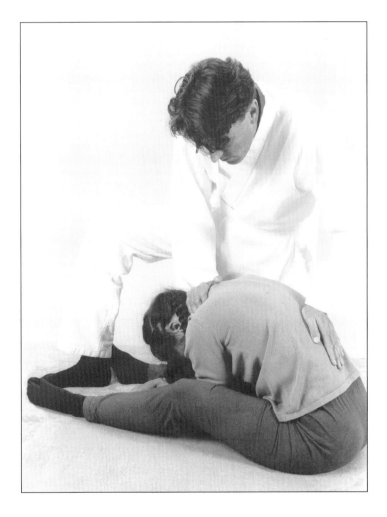

When we're physically active, we're less tense than when we're sitting tensely in a chair, or lying tensely in bed. Movement creates momentum which enables us to perform our activities without tension and without using unnecessary energy.

Breema and Self-Breema release tension, and when we do them correctly, we are more at peace with ourselves. We are in harmony with our activity. The principles that create this harmony can be applied to every activity in our lives.

Anything we do willingly and with interest does not require tension. We do it with the wisdom and dexterity of the body and mind functioning as a unit. That wisdom may even tell us to stop and get the right tool to help us with the activity we are doing.

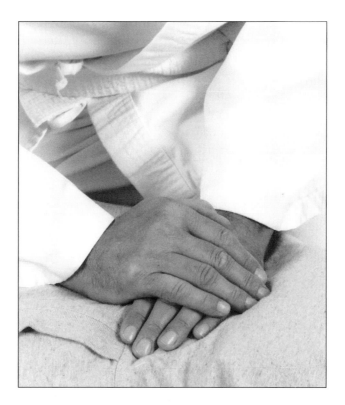

To understand the Universe is very big.
To know yourself is a sufficient inroad!

In order to have less tension, we need some degree of self-knowledge. Then, instead of comparing ourselves to others, or trying to fulfill the images we've unconsciously adopted, we create more reasonable expectations. Breema's principles help us in the direction of becoming familiar with ourselves. The recipient is never dependent on the practitioner's wisdom, but on their own. In the atmosphere of non-judgment that is created, our attitudes and our identification are unnecessary, and we quickly drop them. That's why Breema helps us become free of many levels of tension at once.

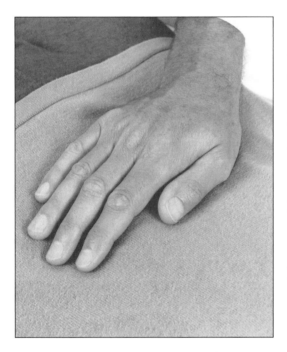

Firmness and Gentleness

Firmness and gentleness are two inseparable qualities. Firmness is firmness with gentleness. Gentleness always has firmness in it. Every contact you make with your partner is both firm and gentle.

Firmness comes from the knowledge that you are connected to your body. Your touch is definite and without hesitation. It's relaxed and conveys the natural weight of your hand and arm. The alive interest of the mind in registering your own body's activity gives you a quality of presence. You are *with* yourself — nowhere else.

Gentleness also comes from your connection to your body. You are receptive, not only to the recipient's body, but to your own body as an energy system. You're sensitive to the support you receive from your connection to your body. This sensitivity is made possible by the participation of the feelings in full receptivity.

Because your aim is to unify your mind, feelings, and body in a common activity, your touch has gentleness. You have a desire for the mind and feelings to participate with you. You stay receptive to feel their presence. This same aim gives your touch firmness. Your hand is on your partner's body for a definite purpose — to support you to know you have a body. The participation of your mind and feelings gives your touch a relaxed quality that is free of tension and force, and at the same time is deeply penetrating.

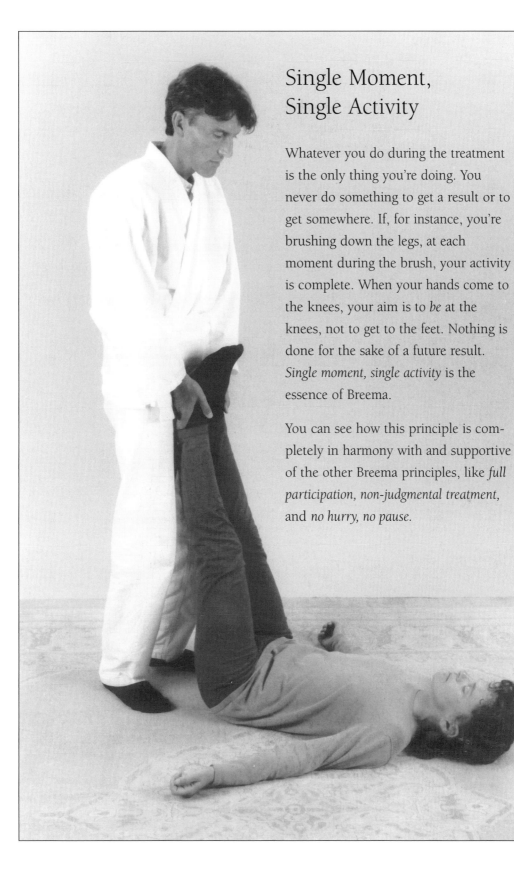

Single Moment, Single Activity

Whatever you do during the treatment is the only thing you're doing. You never do something to get a result or to get somewhere. If, for instance, you're brushing down the legs, at each moment during the brush, your activity is complete. When your hands come to the knees, your aim is to *be* at the knees, not to get to the feet. Nothing is done for the sake of a future result. *Single moment, single activity* is the essence of Breema.

You can see how this principle is completely in harmony with and supportive of the other Breema principles, like *full participation, non-judgmental treatment,* and *no hurry, no pause.*

In Breema, There Is No "Extra"

If you have an "agenda" when you practice, if you want to heal, or even to help, you're not doing Breema. Even if the treatment sequence follows a certain order such as, hold ankles, then hold knees, when I put my hands on the ankles, it's not because I need to move from there up the legs to the knees.

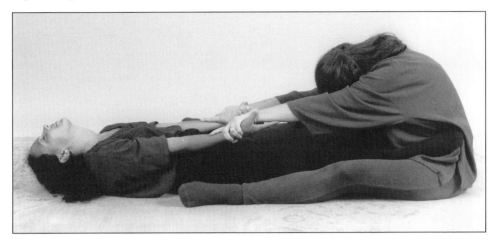

There is *one* body. No matter what part of the body is moving, the whole body is doing the treatment. Of course, there is my body and the recipient's body, but my Consciousness receives the knowledge that there is only *one* Existence, and everything that takes place is an expression of that Existence. When we have this clarity, Breema is a natural activity, and we have no need to think, feel, or sense. While any of these activities may take place, they come and go as "transforming passengers."

The point is to be free from judgment and available to Existence. Then the natural activity of giving or receiving a treatment is in harmony with your nature, and there is no need for "extra."

Waking up means "coming out" of concepts,
*and making a **direct** connection to Existence*
by total disidentification with our mind, feelings, and body.

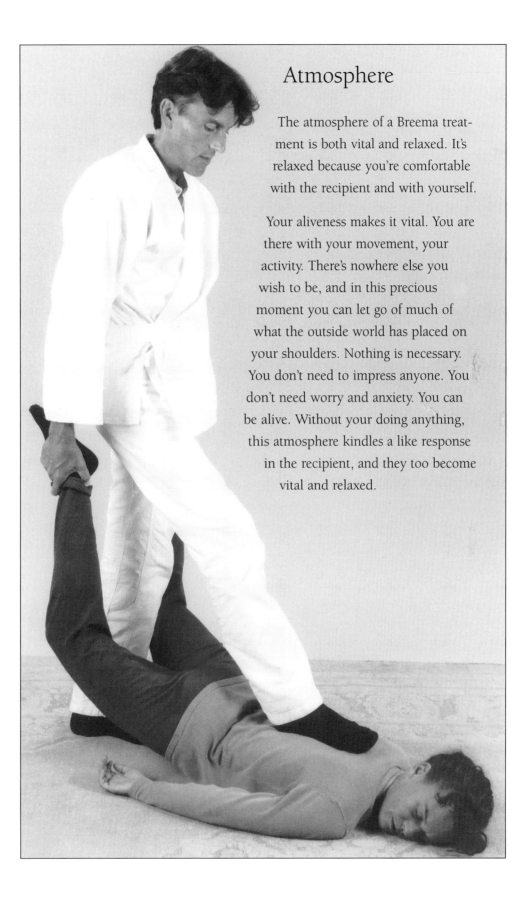

Atmosphere

The atmosphere of a Breema treatment is both vital and relaxed. It's relaxed because you're comfortable with the recipient and with yourself.

Your aliveness makes it vital. You are there with your movement, your activity. There's nowhere else you wish to be, and in this precious moment you can let go of much of what the outside world has placed on your shoulders. Nothing is necessary. You don't need to impress anyone. You don't need worry and anxiety. You can be alive. Without your doing anything, this atmosphere kindles a like response in the recipient, and they too become vital and relaxed.

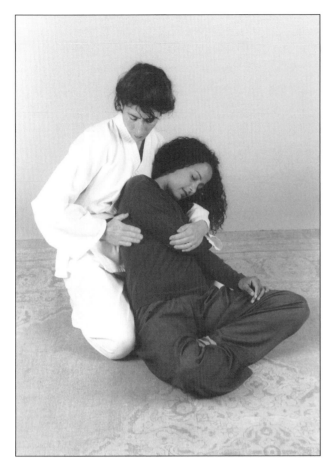

Touch Is a Bridge

Touch is an expression of the desire for Unity. The aim is to bring your total consciousness, in fact, to bring the whole of Existence to your hand when you touch. In that touch, the division between practitioner and recipient disappears.

The principles of gentleness and firmness, and of non-judgment are so important because they create a possibility for that Unity to enter via our touch and fill us up with life.

Touch is a bridge between two fields of energy and their acceptance of each other. *The Breema touch* tunes the emanations of those two energies.

In their Timeless aspect,
the body,
the mind,
and the feelings
are one.

The Aim of Breema Is to Allow Existence to Support You

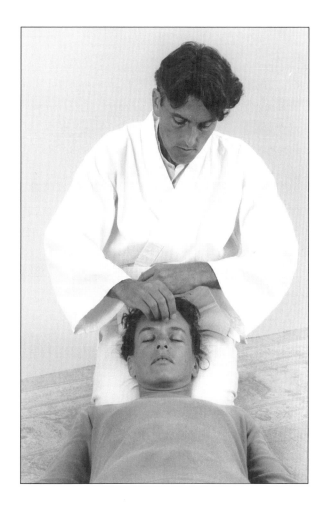

The aim of Breema is to bring you to the level at which you could be nurtured, rather than drained, by your relationship to your body, your surroundings, other people, your feelings, your mind, your life.

If we remember that our aim is to be nurtured, we let go, perhaps for the first time, of our judgment of others. This non-judgment has a taste of freedom in it, because it includes letting go of self-judgment.

When we become free of judgment, we become *receptive* to the harmonizing nature of Existence. Our mind becomes receptive, and gives us clarity. Our feelings become receptive, and give us presence. Our body becomes receptive, and is vital and available.

The atmosphere created by the practitioner's openness to life during the treatment affects the recipient directly, because, in truth, practitioner and recipient are two manifestations of one energy, one life, one Unified Field of Existence, which is both the Source of all creation and that creation itself.

How to Choose a Treatment

At first, while your repertoire is limited, you'll need to choose from among the treatments you've recently learned in class when practicing with your partner. Once your repertoire has expanded a bit, you can practice the treatments that your body especially feels like doing. By doing what *your* body enjoys, the recipient receives exactly what he or she needs most. By allowing your body to choose the treatment, you'll find that naturally the recipient receives what you wish to do, and what you do is what the recipient wishes to receive. In the energy field that is created between practitioner and recipient, communication is precise, continuous, and non-verbal.

At the same time, your commonsense wisdom will tell you if a particular treatment isn't appropriate for the recipient because of certain health conditions (for instance, osteoporosis, dislocated shoulder, etc.). If your mind comes in and questions whether or not a particular treatment can be safely practiced with the recipient, consider choosing a different treatment. You will find many other opportunities to practice the first one. Also, when you're unsure, there's nothing wrong with checking to make sure the recipient is comfortable by asking them. Talking is a form of exchange too, and is constructive. Of course, as you become more advanced, verbal checking is less necessary.

Every Breema treatment, no matter how simple, contains enough food for a lifetime of practice. You can never become too advanced for a particular treatment. No matter how dexterous you are, there is always room to apply every principle more fully.

Because even the simplest Breema treatment is complete by itself, there really is no need to try to change any treatment. Once you've had at least several years of intensive experience as a practitioner, it is appropriate to allow your body to improvise during a treatment.

You're not really improvising, because when the body's instinctive wisdom guides you, whatever you do is Breema. The instinctive wisdom of the body receives an *impression*, a *taste*, at the presence of Awareness and Consciousness. That taste allows the body to move with the support and guidance of Existence. This understanding may lead you to an even greater understanding — ultimately, Breema is not a method. It is a natural and harmonious response to Existence that allows the natural wisdom of the body to manifest.

The treatments, although diverse in form, are all based on the same underlying principles. Different treatments can be practiced sequentially to make a longer "session." Maintain contact with the recipient between sequences, and bow at the end of your final module. Nothing begins, nothing ends. What *is* is *present*.

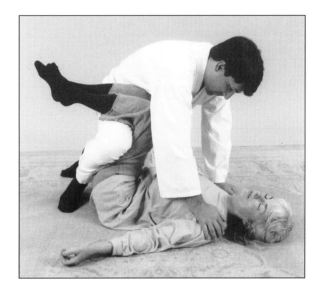

Recognizing that we are "asleep"
*and **waking up** from it*
is the meaning of "I exist."

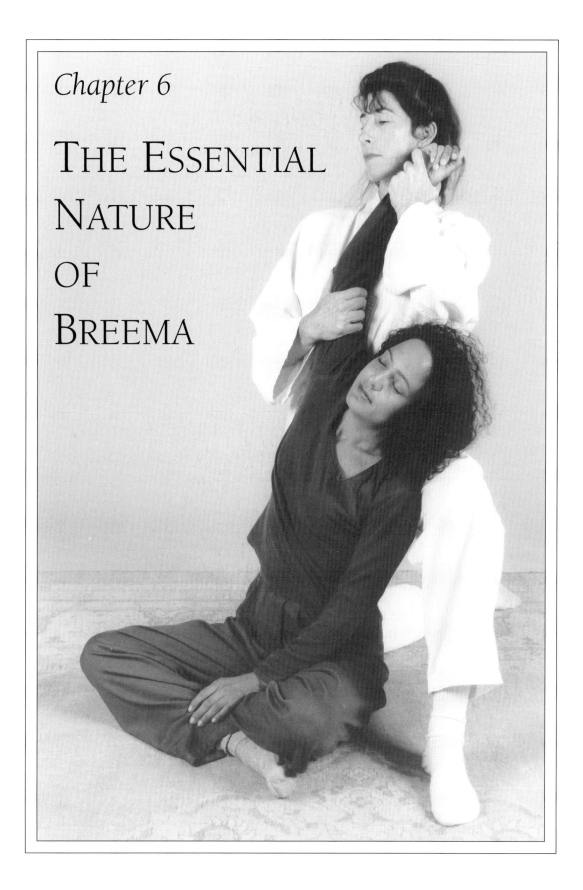

Chapter 6

THE ESSENTIAL
NATURE
OF
BREEMA

Breema is a natural expression of Existence.

THE ESSENTIAL NATURE OF BREEMA

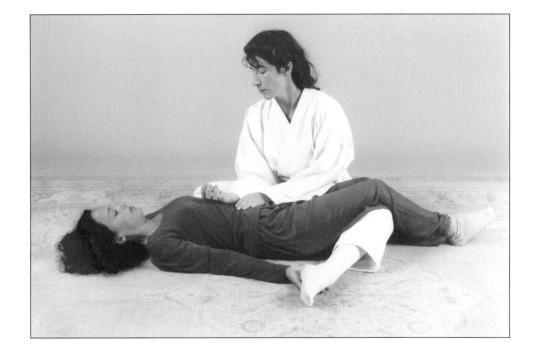

Working with Breema Principles in Daily Life

One night, Malichek and I were cooking dinner together. I was sautéing sliced onions over a high flame, hurriedly stirring and patting them with a wooden spoon. Malichek watched me for a moment, then said, "Jon, you see how you're doing it?" Immediately, I felt the unpleasantly nervous quality of my movements, which came from a self-imposed sense of urgency. Malichek took the spoon and leisurely stirred the onions in a wide circular motion that involved his whole body, and swept all the onions to one side of the pan. Then with one broad back-handed stroke, he spread the onions evenly over the whole pan. That was

Breema! Although I considered myself a good cook, I saw that there was more to cooking than I had realized. There is an energy exchange between me and the ingredients as I prepare and cook them that leaves an imprint on the food, like the spices I use to flavor it. Moreover, the way I am *while* cooking — the state of my mind, feelings, and body, and the degree of harmony between them — is in itself a meal that I'm eating moment by moment.

In a few seconds, Malichek had shown me the meaning of bringing Breema into my daily life. Every moment, we are exchanging life energy with the people, plants, animals, and objects around us. Breema principles can be applied anywhere, anytime, from *body comfortable* to *full and harmonious participation of mind and feelings in the activity of the body*.

Every activity of the body could be enjoyed. It's possible to stir onions as though giving them a treatment. Breema could expand from a method of treatment to a daily practice of creating harmony and balance.

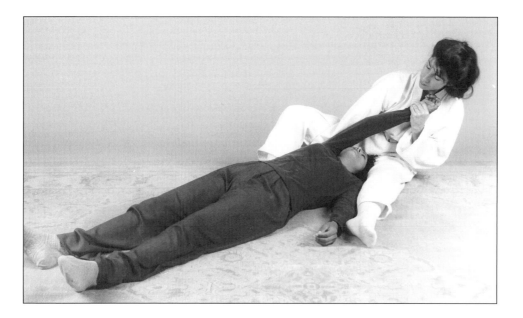

"I exist" is a new territory of Consciousness,
above our thoughts and feelings.
*In fact, this **I** is given*
in the absence of thoughts and feelings.

Breema and the Feelings

We do not know our true feelings, but we do know how to nurture them. When our mind and body work as a unit, and in harmony with each other, we clear the ground for this nurturing process to take place. Then many things support and nurture our feelings.

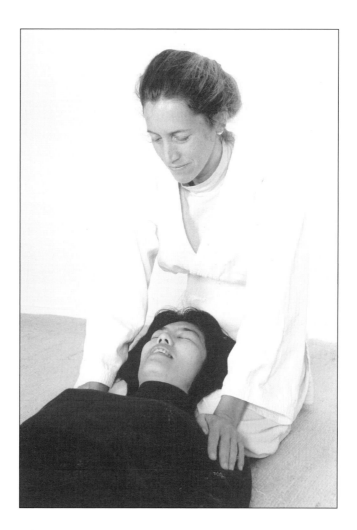

Our feelings are nurtured:

When we are *present* in our daily activities,

When we are less judgmental,

When we have acceptance of ourselves and the people around us,

When we do things with attention and use our abilities to their maximum,

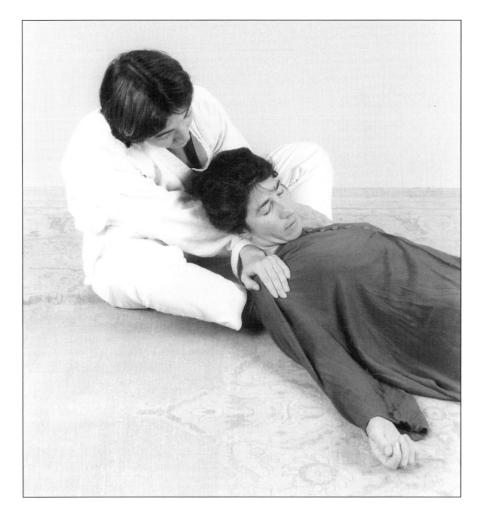

When we willingly do something that needs to be done,

When we make ourselves available to the needs of our friends and neighbors,

When we have a sense of a greater Existence than ourselves, and in our actions and activities we carry that sense with us,

When we practice kindness and forgiveness,

When we wish not to think negatively about the people we come in contact with,

When we allow the simple pleasures of life to be fully appreciated,

When we live our life with gratitude for that which is given to us,

When we acknowledge that we are being helped by what's been set up in our surroundings,

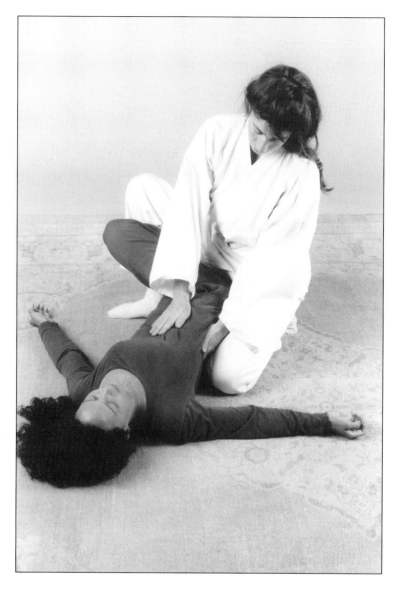

When we remember how dear our parents are, and how much we owe to them,

When we wish to support everyone we're supported by,

When we acknowledge and respect the good deeds of others,

When we are willing to pay for what we receive,

When we have a sense of gratitude for our daily accomplishments,

When we appreciate that which is, and have well-wishing for better,

When our words and thoughts about others are sincere,

When we train ourselves to do small things for the welfare of our planet and humanity,

When we use things correctly and avoid misusing them,

When we shake hands with a friend while connected to our body,

When our mind is receptive while listening,

When we appreciate nourishment more than stimulation,

When we wish to take good care of ourselves, simply and effectively,

When we don't take advantage of the misfortune of others,

When we remember the temporariness of the life of the body,

When we relate to each occasion as if it's the only time we have,

When we live each day as if it's the only day we have left to live,

When we live less and less in our mind, and recognize that we're surrounded by life,

When we appreciate the good in others, and see their shortcomings simply as a lack of knowledge and experience in some particular area, rather than as faults,

When we have room to see opposing sides at the same time,

When we have a small goal to accomplish each day and we have well-wishing for ourselves to accomplish it,

When we remember that life has meaning,

When we wish this meaning to reveal itself to us,

When we pray non-verbally,

When our posture towards life is humble and has dignity,

When we say "yes" and when we say "no," not out of weakness, but from our knowing,

When we look at money as energy and energy as money, and we economize wisely,

When we treat others as we wish to be treated,

When we respect others' belongings and accomplishments and have well-wishing for them,

When we respect simplicity more than complication,

When we wish to say that which we know, and avoid saying what we don't know.

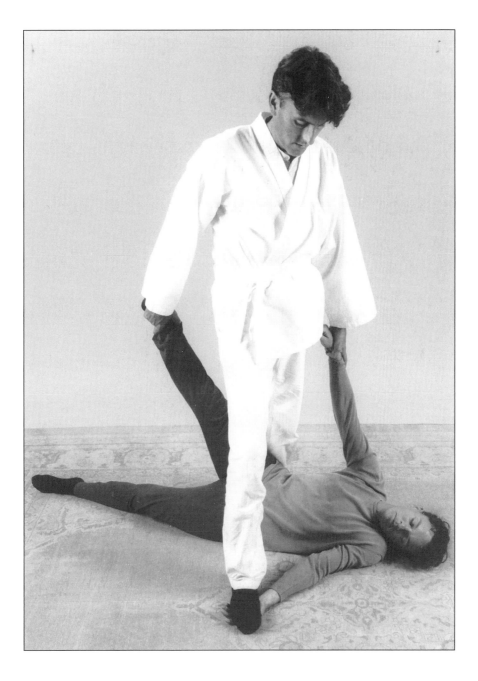

Emotional Energy

Emotional energy is like a spring. When someone is disturbed, their waters are stirred up and muddy.

We don't need to have any judgment about it. We know their spring is disturbed, and that it's going to settle. We don't have to deal with their disturbance specifically — it's going to settle naturally.

The best support for their spring to settle is a non-judgmental treatment.

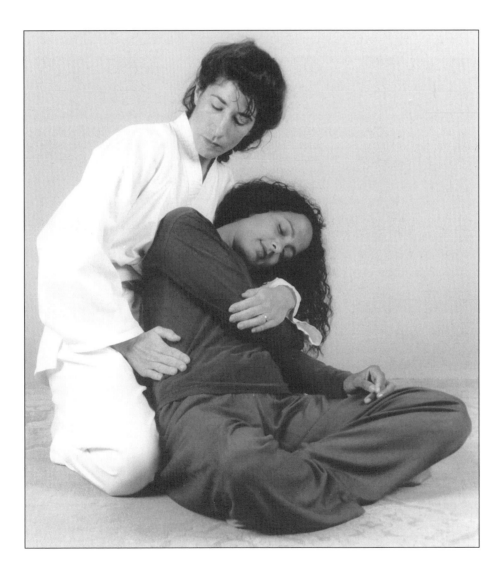

The Light of Acceptance

People remember past unpleasant events, and they suffer with their memories. We can help, not by suppressing or ignoring these memories, but by bringing them into the light of acceptance. We need to understand that the body that experienced that trauma no longer exists. Every cell has been recycled and remade. The part of us that relives our emotional reaction and suffers because of it, is really only a minor part of us. Our essential Self cannot be damaged by the actions of others, because it is free of memory. That which is brought to the present and seen for what it is, in the light of acceptance and in the absence of judgment, is a shortcut to healing the past.

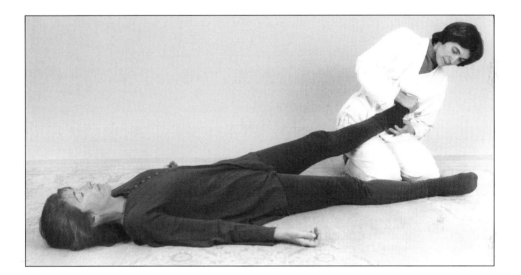

We are constantly taking in impressions without "digesting" them fully.
That's why we can't help living in the past.
We rehash our experiences because they have not been digested properly.
Connection to the body, in its true sense, is in the direction of finding something within us
that can digest impressions as they are received.

Healing

The essence of all healing is in understanding. To be able to heal yourself, you have to understand yourself. This understanding begins simply. The first step is to actively register that you have a body. Of course, you know that theoretically, but this knowledge is not alive and present with you during your day. Seeing that you live without this basic knowledge is the first indication that you are not who you believe you are.

Slowly, by seeing this, the person who believes he knows himself and who believes he is someone important, becomes less self-important. The less self-important you are, the less you are affected by how other people think of you, and the less you are afraid of people. You no longer try to make people believe you are something you are not. You are no longer so dependent on receiving admiration.

Most sickness is the result of disharmony between the mind and feelings. Our desires create conflict in us which brings about this disharmony.

Healing is the process of creating peace. We heal by accepting our illness without fear, without translating pain into suffering. The instinctive nature of our body, when it receives support from the feelings, naturally emanates healing energy. By making our mind comfortable, this healing energy is able to manifest. Then we are attracted to the people, foods, medicines, and conditions that help us heal.

When we are connected to the knowledge of "I have a body," we manifest with more vital force. We waste less energy and accomplish more. When we're relaxed, balanced, and available, we have a different posture and attitude towards what we're doing. Even chores, necessary activities we may not particularly like, can be done with willing energy which doesn't invite conflict. When we do something willingly, we benefit, because our mind, feelings, and body function harmoniously, and gain more dexterity in the process. We experience a sense of fulfillment. This willing participation in our activities is also a form of healing, because it results in greater vitality.

*In the imaginery state of sleep, our I-ego bases all its actions on false perceptions and separateness. Our **I-Consciousness** knows Existence is one unified whole.*

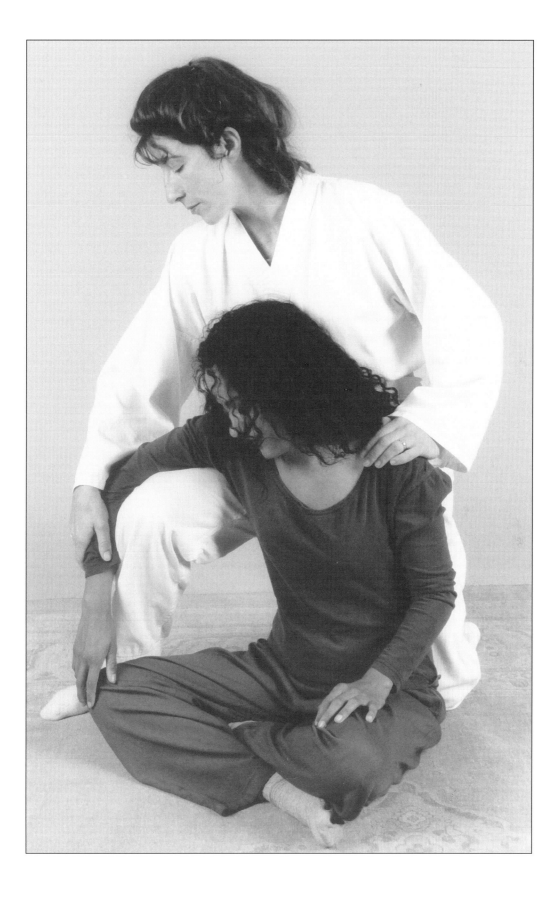

Breema and the Mind

In order to verify the truth of what we think, we need the assistance of our feelings and our body. That which we think must also be felt and sensed simultaneously.

We support this process by giving the mind one simple job to do, asking it to receptively *register* our own body's weight and breathing.

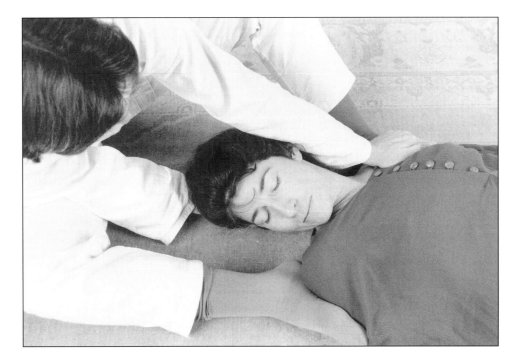

At first, we find this challenging — our mind has long been accustomed to being our "boss." It repeatedly wants to return to its world of imagination and useless wandering, and shuffle and reshuffle the information it has received from the outside, falsely labeling it as knowledge and sometimes even as understanding. This misuse of the meaning of knowledge and understanding keeps us more at the periphery of the mind, and invites our mechanicality to further dominate us.

Partial knowledge is complex.
Total knowledge is simple.
The person who has real understanding is very simple.
The person with partial understanding is complicated.

So whenever we recognize that we are again lost in our thoughts, we simply ask our mind to return to its new job and remain with it until we experience the presence of a new energy which we call *Being-presence*. Then, once again, our three aspects are actively participating in life.

Slowly, we become familiar with the distinctive "taste" that's present when our mind is registering the body at the presence of the feelings. These are not the "feelings" we are familiar with, which work only via attraction and repulsion. These true feelings are simply *present*.

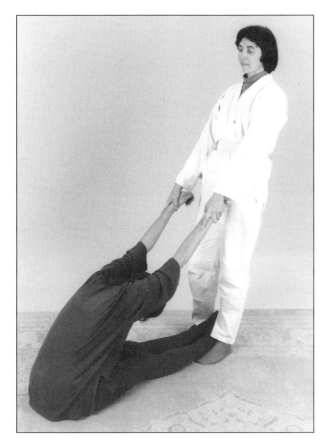

This is our direction. The mind does not *think* about the body's weight and breath, it *registers* the body's weight and breathing. This registration is the receptive quality of mind that we are after — it takes place in the *absence* of thought. When the mind is receptive, we *experience* that which it registers. When our feelings also participate receptively, we sense and feel that which the mind registers. When mind, feelings, and body all experience the fact of "there is a body," our experience becomes more definite knowledge, and we have less identification. Then, when we have essential questions, questions about the purpose and meaning of our lives, we have a base. Instead of entertaining these questions abstractly, we may seek knowledge that we can verify through our actual experience, through "taste," rather than settling for theories to believe in.

Once our mind "settles into" a correct relationship with the feelings and the body, it could, with their support, think intentionally, ponder, and reason soundly. That's why our aim is to bring the mind, feelings, and body to work together.

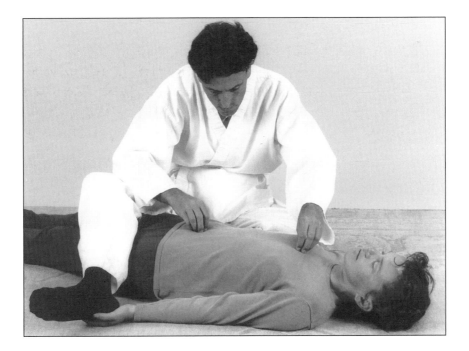

I once asked Malichek what he thought about Teachings.
"Respect all Teachings," he told me,
"but follow only that which you can verify for yourself."

The Treatment Needs No Philosophy

Consciousness allows us to see things as they are,
and in that, there is no room for thought.

Breema is not a path, not a "way to" anywhere. When you do Breema, the aim is to simply do Breema, not to understand something.

The physical principles of Breema are all you need to be occupied with during a treatment: registering your body's breathing, experiencing that your body has weight, using your whole body, keeping your body comfortable, supporting your partner's body, and allowing their body to support you. These principles bring you right to your activity, and help you to be constantly more present, to participate more fully in the treatment. They make you simpler, not more complicated.

The Breema treatment and principles help you become *natural*. The principles are not philosophical. Breema is the expression of natural laws. When you do Breema, you don't want to know *about* anything. Your aim is to *directly* know "I have a body." This knowing is *experienced* as "connection to the body," which means body moves naturally, mind registers the body's movement receptively, and the feelings support this activity with calm, joyful presence. In other words, you are not elsewhere. Body, mind, and feelings are present and participating in harmony with each other, in the activity of the treatment. This needs no philosophy.

The more alive your practice is, the greater its decrystallizing influence on your body, mind, and feelings. This, in turn, increases the possibility that this philosophy could touch you, awakening and nurturing your desire for understanding. But you need not worry about this process. There is a saying, "The tree ripens the fruit. Do you think you have to concern yourself with how it does it? When the fruit is ripe, you will know it. And if you don't, the tree will tell you by letting the fruit fall to the ground."

Your mind and feelings are just an open space when you do Breema. If that space is filled by receiving a realization during the treatment, wonderful. You're welcome to enjoy it. But don't search for realizations. In fact, desire-less activity is what Breema really is.

There is a spring within us, and it's connected to the Universal reservoir of the Field of Existence. Of course there's communication and exchange between the spring and the reservoir, but it takes place naturally, and doesn't need your desire. The vitality you feel after giving a treatment is a function of the spring. Breema is the simplest form of natural body movement, yet during the treatment, you receive exactly what you need. Everything the treatment accomplishes is the result of the life force passing through our body in its natural rhythm, in harmony with everything that is. That harmony is already there. You don't need to make it your goal or desire. Be simple — do Breema and enjoy it. That's all.

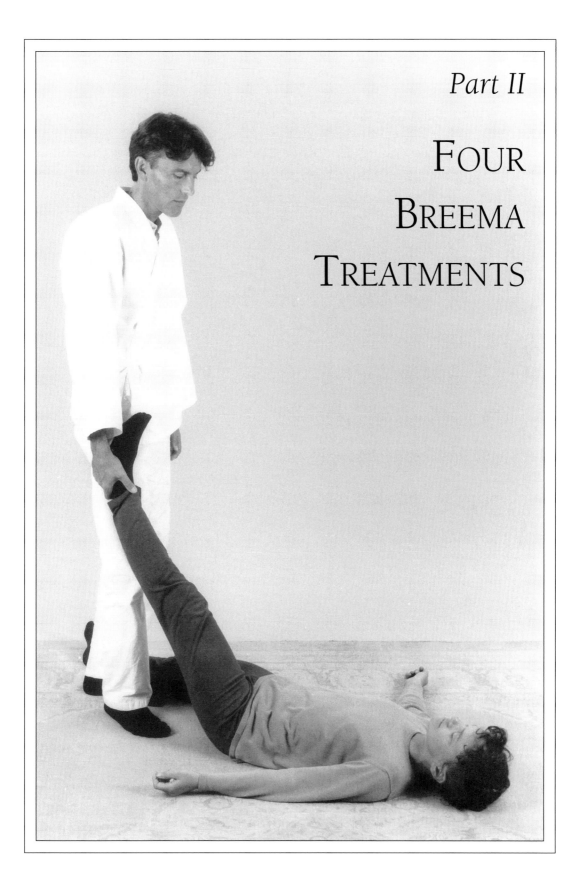

Part II

FOUR
BREEMA
TREATMENTS

The mind doesn't tell the body
how to do a Breema treatment.
It may tell you what move comes next,
but not how to do it.

INTRODUCTION TO THE TREATMENTS

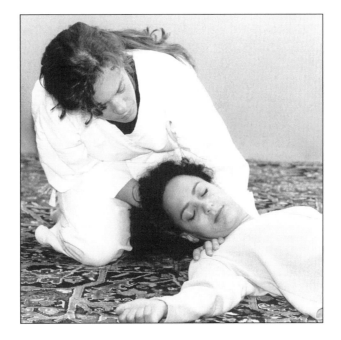

Learning with the Body

There is an art to learning Breema. You need three things:

1. Receptivity.

2. Registration of the body's weight and breath.

3. Sincerity.

If you apply these three things, you will learn Breema well, and the process of learning will be very rewarding.

When you're in class, be receptive and relaxed. Take an impression of the treatment that the instructor is demonstrating. Don't worry about memorizing. With enough repetition, you will make the treatment a part of yourself. While you're practicing, let yourself again receive an impression — see how the treatment is affecting *you*. Trust your own experience, and go with it. When your practice is nourishing, you are going in the right direction. That experience is valuable to you, and you'll wish to have more experiences. Your appetite for Breema will grow, and your practice will stay alive!

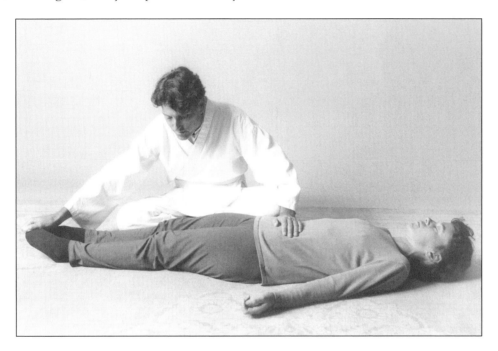

You don't learn Breema sequences with your mind. You look at the sequence with your body, mind, and feelings, and then all three do it together. Your mind doesn't learn the sequence; all of you does.

If your body, mind, and feelings learn the treatment, then you learn it exactly. If your mind learns it, it may remember the form of the sequence precisely, but it doesn't remember the feeling and sensation of the treatment. The experience of the body and feelings are not a part of that memory.

That's why, when you study Breema, you need interest, sincerity, and presence. Your mind is attentive, and because it's registering your body's weight and breath, it remains receptive, instead of tensing with the effort of concentration. Your body remains relaxed and available. Your feelings add the qualities of interest, sincerity, and presence. This way, you learn not only the form of Breema — the unified activity of your body, mind, and feelings enables you to receive an impression of the *atmosphere* of the treatment, which is the most important part.

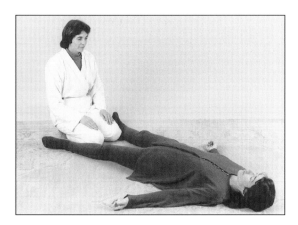

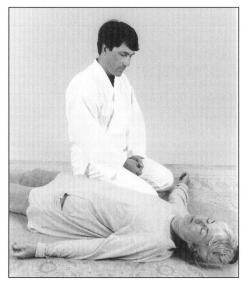

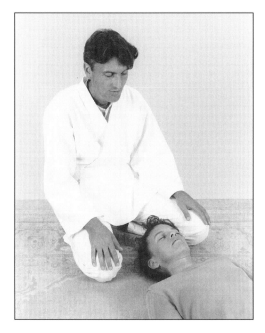

Before You Touch Your Partner's Body

Allow your body to be comfortable.

Drop your shoulders.

Experience the weight of your body on the ground.

Allow your body to have a slight motion to the right and to the left just to remind you: body has weight and is breathing.

Sit or stand as though you are alone and just breathe.

Experience the effects of inhalation on your abdomen and upper body, then experience the effects of exhalation on the abdomen and lower body.

"Collecting yourself" by coming to the body prepares you for the treatment so that your initial contact with the recipient's body is Breema. This preparation is not really time-dependent. It's possible to do it in a single inhalation and exhalation.

Before you touch the recipient's body, you have to pay respect by carrying two things with you — the knowledge that your own body breathes and the knowledge that body has weight. Respect means to accept without pre-conditions, without judgment. When the mind registers weight and breath, it is free of judgment.

DEEPENING THE CONNECTION TO THE BODY

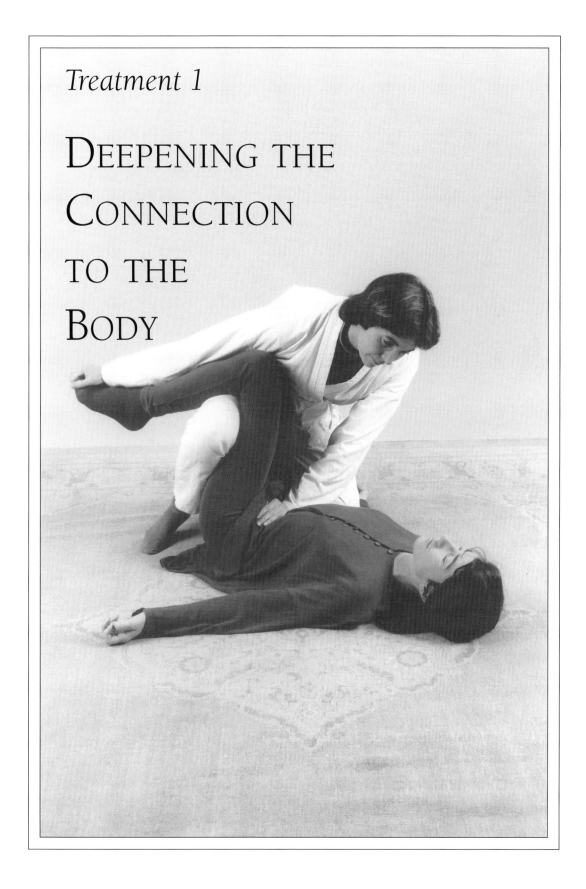

Treatment Steps

✧ *Sit comfortably in seiza (kneeling) position at recipient's feet.*

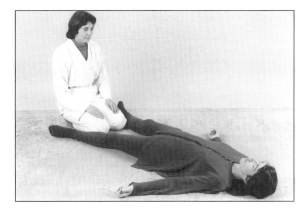

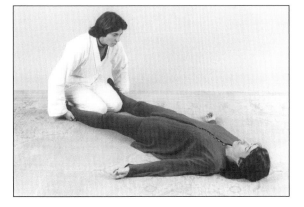

✧ *Slide your hands under recipient's heels and lean back, using your whole body to bring recipient's feet onto your lap, with the soles of their feet against your abdomen.*

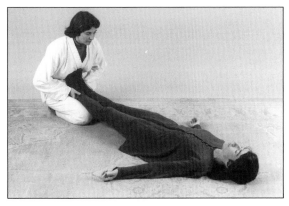

✧ *Slide your hands to recipient's knees.*

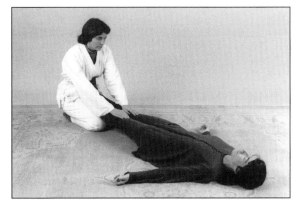

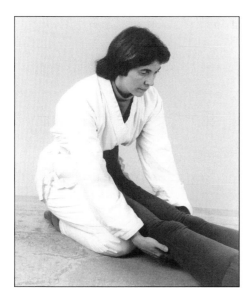

✧ *Staying connected with your partner, slide your hands to hold under knees, and come up onto your knees. Your abdomen naturally supports their feet, and your hands support below their knees.*

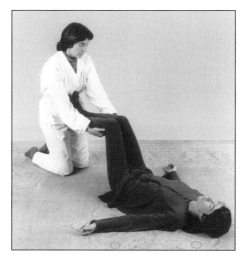

✧ *Lean forward, bringing the recipient's legs towards their abdomen as your hands slide from under to on top of the knees — again staying connected with your partner.*

✧ *Hold for 3 breaths.*

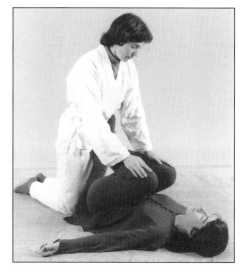

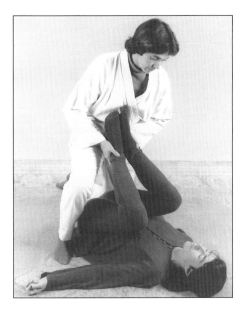

❖ Come to kneeling on your left knee at recipient's right side with your right foot sole-flat-on-floor, and drape recipient's legs over your right thigh.

❖ Hold abdomen with left hand and toes of both feet with right hand for 3 breaths.

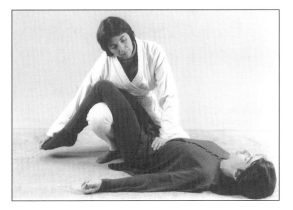

❖ Rotate (circle) your body 3 times clockwise (lean forward, right, back, left), then 3 times counterclockwise (lean forward, left, back, right), still holding abdomen and toes.

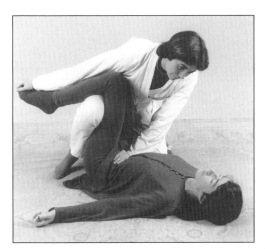

❖ Lean into the chest near the shoulders for one full breath. (See facing page.)

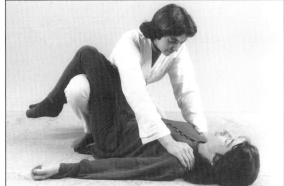

Working on the Chest

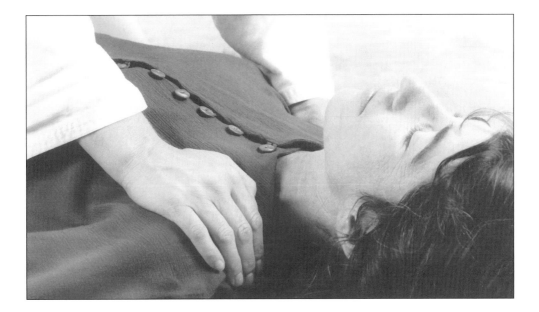

Many Breema treatments and Self-Breema exercises work with the upper part of the chest, in the area on both the right and left sides just below the collarbone, just inward from the shoulder joint. Each side includes an area about the size of your palm.

When this area is free of tension, the body's posture is more in harmony with nature, and we find it easier to move with our natural rhythm. Breema treatments hold, tap, brush, and lean into the upper chest in a variety of rhythms and intensities. When our hands are placed correctly on the chest, we can lean in with our whole body weight without causing any discomfort. On the contrary, a tremendous letting go of tension in the upper back is often experienced by both practitioner and recipient. If your hands are positioned in just the right place, you experience the joy of a "perfect fit" — the upper chest seems a natural template for the contour of your palms.

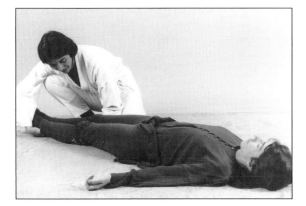

✧ Lower recipient's legs to floor,
   supporting under knees with your
   left forearm and hand, and under
   both heels with your right hand.

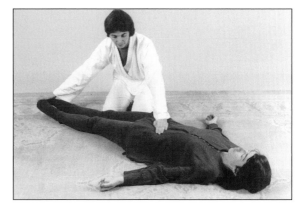

✧ Hold abdomen and toes for 3
   breaths.

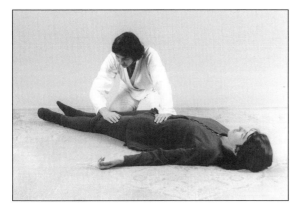

✧ Keeping left hand on abdomen,
   brush with your right hand from
   abdomen down recipient's left leg
   to toes and off, 3 times.

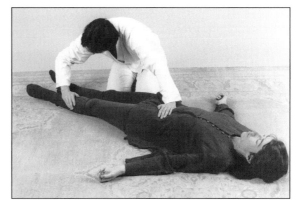

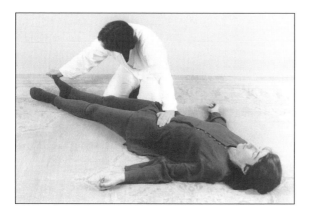

✧ *Then, brush from abdomen down right leg to toes and off, 3 times.*

✧ *Hold abdomen with your left hand for one breath.*

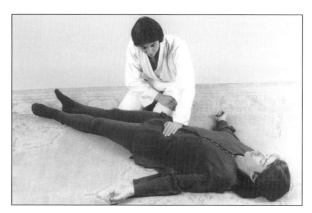

✧ *Release and bow.*

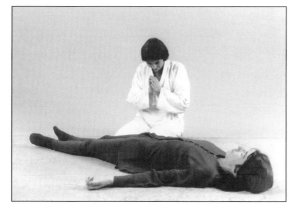

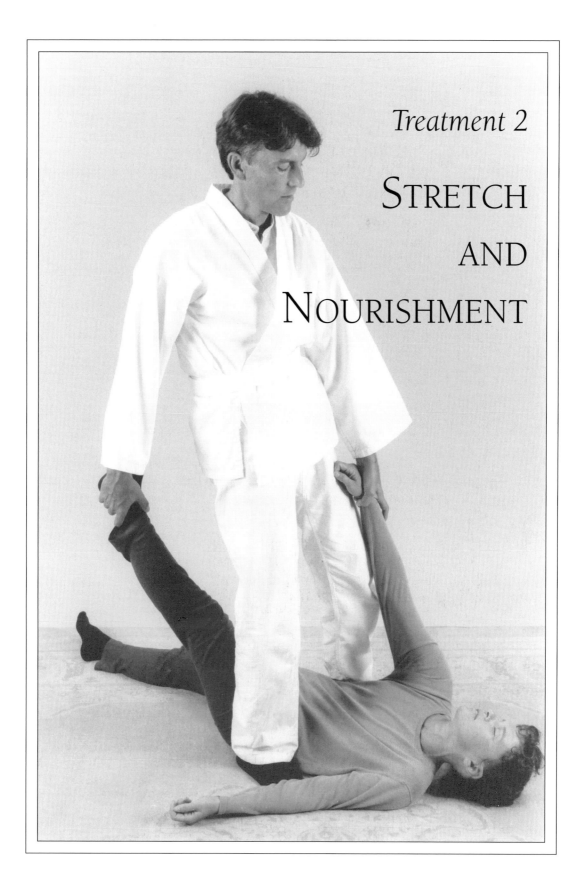

Treatment 2

STRETCH

AND

NOURISHMENT

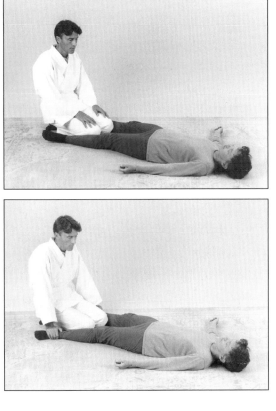

Treatment Steps

✧ *Sit in seiza position at feet.*

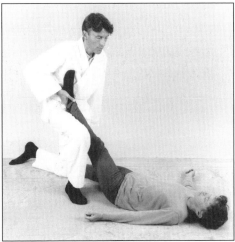

✧ *Hold insteps for 3 breaths.*

✧ *Using your whole body, stand up, lifting left leg under heel.*

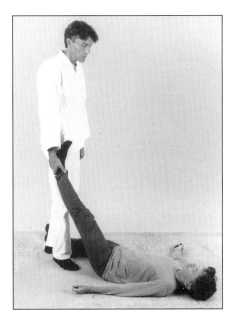

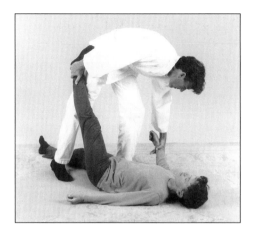

✧ *Then lift right forearm, by holding just above the wrist and extending your forefinger along the forearm.*

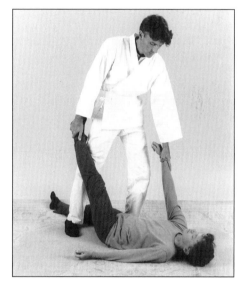

✧ *Shifting your weight to the left, step your right foot from between recipient's legs...*

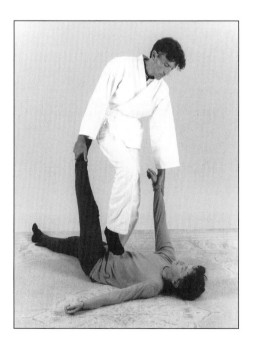

✧ *...over the abdomen and to the floor by their left hip. Your left foot stays at recipient's right side.*

✧ *Shift your weight from foot to foot, alternately stretching arm and leg rhythmically, letting your whole body participate.*

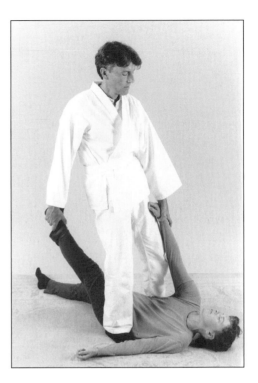

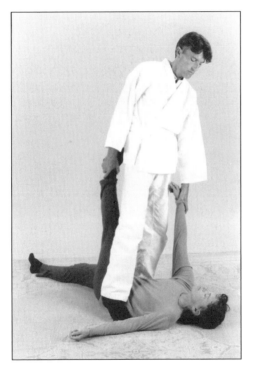

Continue for 3 breaths.

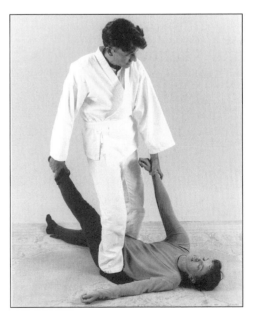

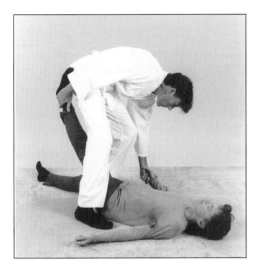

✦ *Slowly lower arm to the floor as you walk backward.*

✦ *Step your right foot to between recipient's legs, continuing to walk backward, lowering leg to the floor.*

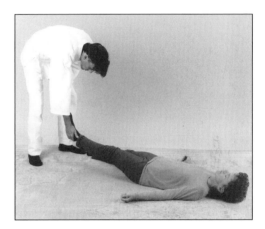

✦ *Repeat the sequence on pages 139–141, holding right leg and left forearm.*

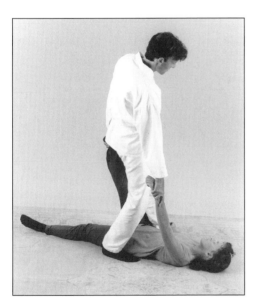

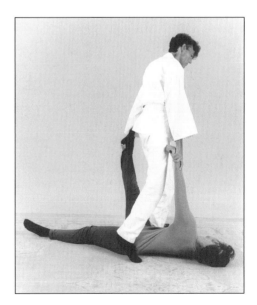

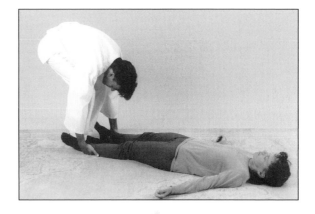

✧ *Lift both legs by heels.*

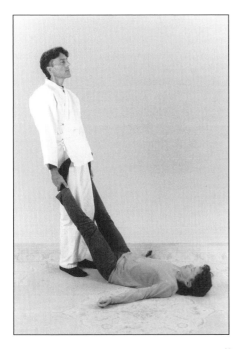

✧ *Letting recipient's feet rest at your sides, lean back, stretching legs.*

✧ *Slowly come forward, releasing the stretch, and bringing the recipient's feet together in front of you.*

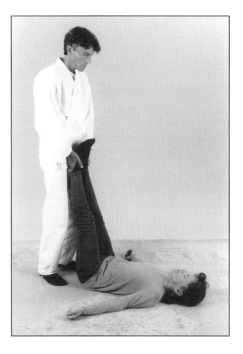

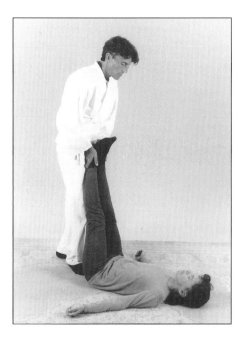

✧ *Still holding legs upright, walk clockwise in a small circle, thus moving recipient's feet and legs in a small circle.*

Make two more circles, then switch directions, walking counterclockwise 3 times (recipient's feet stay together).

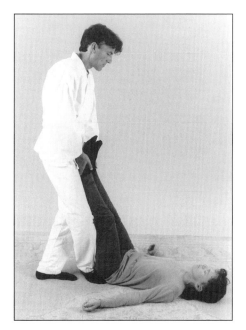

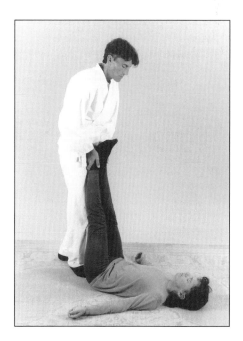

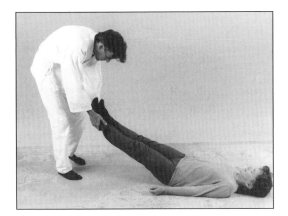

❖ Walk backwards, slowly lowering
legs to floor. Let your own body
rock from side to side with the
natural momentum of each step,
so your arms and the recipient's
legs swing gently side to side.

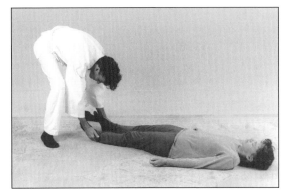

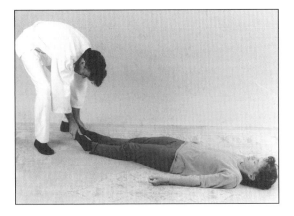

❖ Brush hands off tops of feet.

❖ Release and bow.

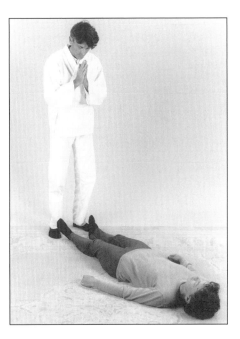

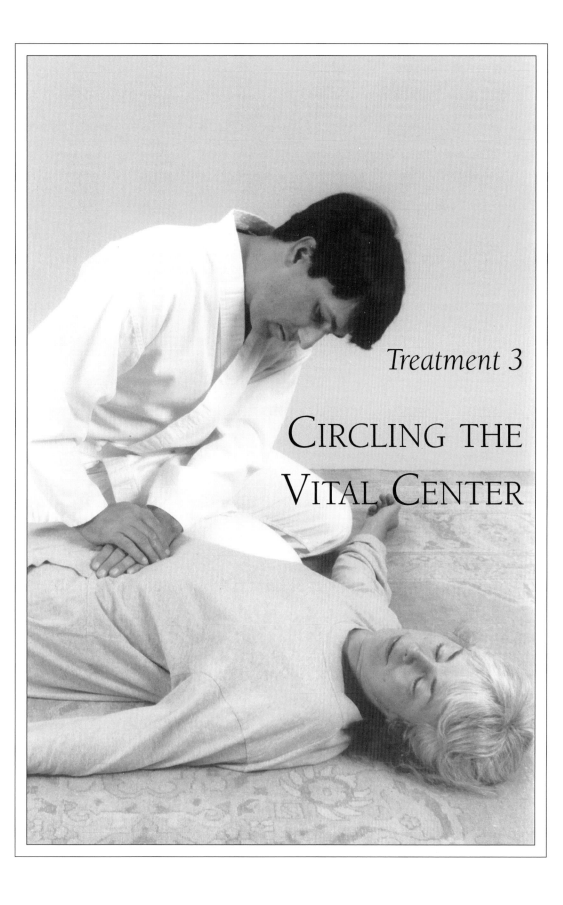

Treatment 3

CIRCLING THE VITAL CENTER

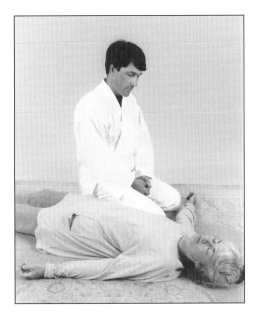

Treatment Steps

✧ *Sit comfortably (in either seiza or cross-legged position) at recipient's right side.*

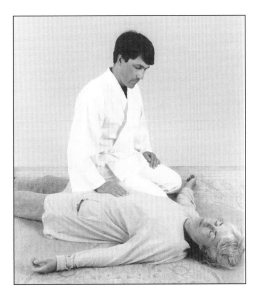

✧ *Place your right hand on abdomen (your fingertips are oriented towards recipient's head).*

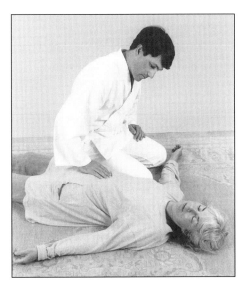

✧ *Keeping your hand "in place," rotate so that the weight of your body shifts in a clockwise circle, which, in turn, shifts the emphasis of your weight around the perimeter of your hand in a clockwise circle 3 times.*

Emphasis — Not Pressure

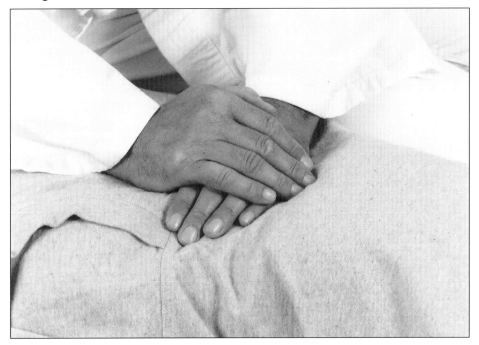

Emphasis means that the weight of your body goes to where you are leaning. There is a big difference between "emphasis" and "pressure." Pressure is determined by measurement, and comes from the mind. Emphasis comes from receptivity, and is the naturally established communication between two bodies.

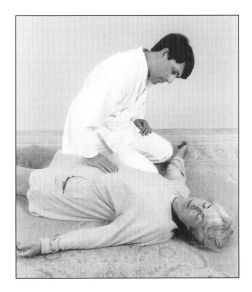
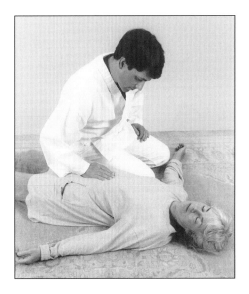

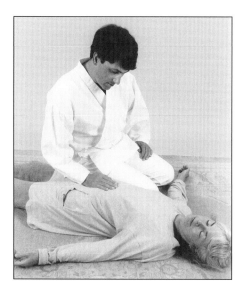

❖ *Repeat, now rotating counterclockwise 3 times.*

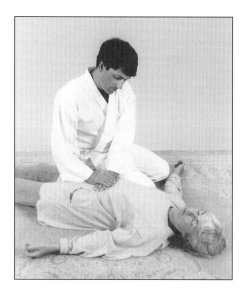

❖ *Slide your left hand (palm-down) underneath your right hand (and perpendicular to your right hand) so your fingers are oriented towards recipient's left side.*

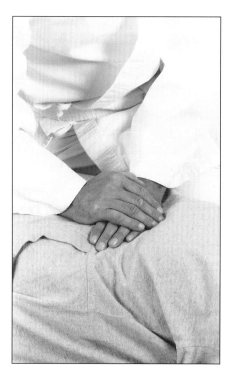

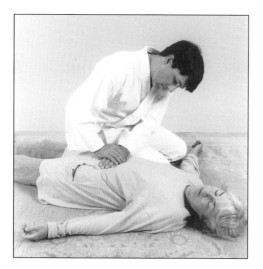

✧ Rotate, shifting the emphasis of your weight clockwise several times, then counterclockwise several times.

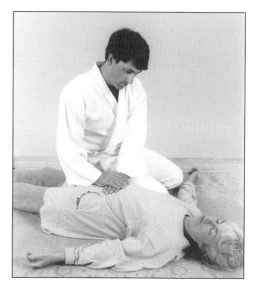

✧ Hold your hands in this position for 3 breaths.

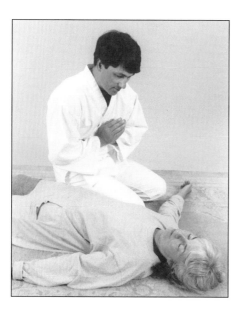

✧ Release and bow.

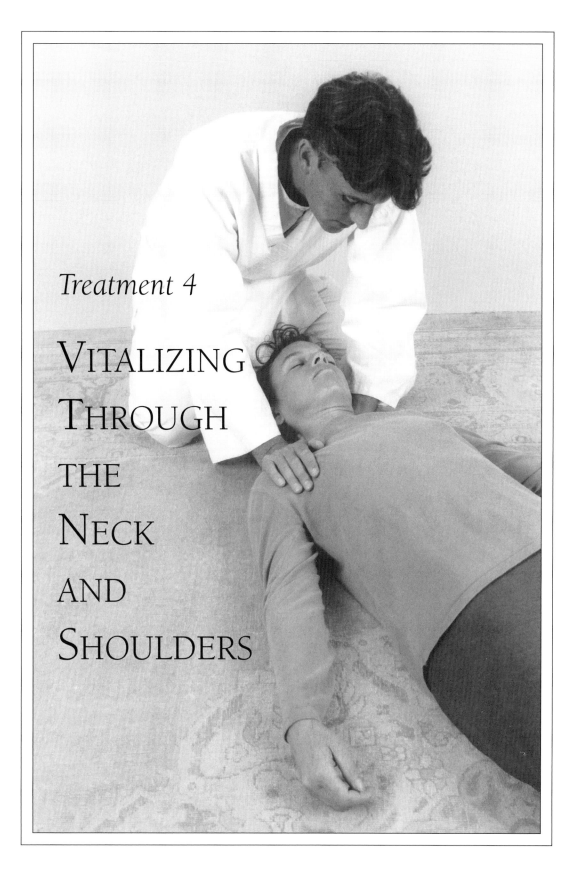

Treatment 4

VITALIZING
THROUGH
THE
NECK
AND
SHOULDERS

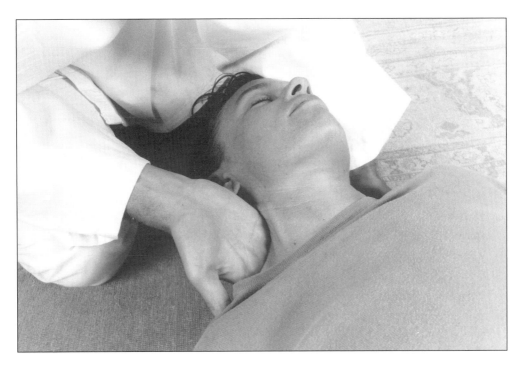

Working on the Neck and Head

The neck and head are particularly sensitive areas of the body. When working with the head and neck, it's very important that your hands be warm. If your hands are cold, hold them under warm water before starting the treatment, or work first on the lower body, which is less temperature-sensitive, until your hands warm up. As a rule, it's best to begin your treatments at the feet, so that the recipient relaxes and opens up. By the time you're ready to work with the upper body, they've learned to trust your touch and can be more fully receptive.

Your emphasis should be on moving gradually and working gently. It's always better to "err" on the side of gentleness. Never try to *force* the recipient's neck to move into a specific position or through a particular range of motion. At the same time, give respect to the head and neck by touching them as naturally as you'd pet a cat, recognizing that all parts of the body are just body, just soil. In other words, what's needed to safely and successfully do Breema at the head and neck is to be especially tuned in to the principles. Simple *presence* is needed, nothing less, nothing more. With that as your base, the treatment is pure joy.

Treatment Steps

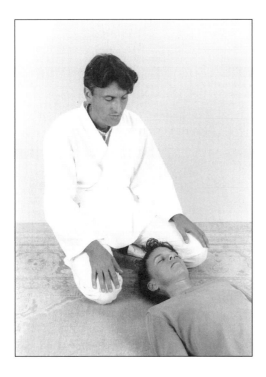

✧ *Sit in seiza position at head.*

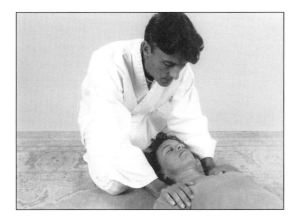

✧ *Lean forward and hold shoulders for 3 breaths.*

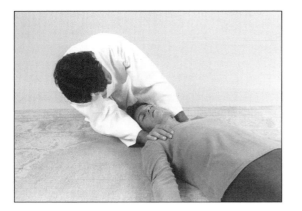

✧ *Lean alternately into the shoulders, keeping your center of gravity low (recipient's shoulders should move towards their feet).*

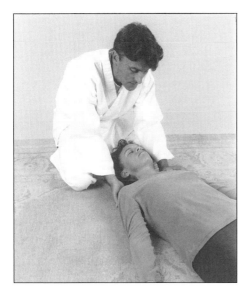

✧ Slide hands, palms up, under shoulders, so their shoulder blades rest in your palms. (The photograph below illustrates the placement of your hands on the recipient's back.)

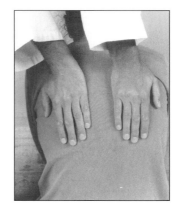

✧ Alternately, lean back slightly, then down and to the right, then back again, then down and to the left several times (so your body moves in a figure 8). As your body leans, your hands gradually and naturally move in increments from the shoulder blades towards the neck.

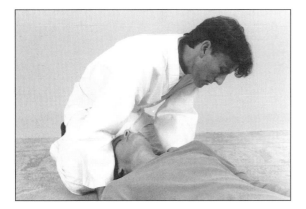

✧ When you reach the neck, continue the same movement and rhythm with fingertips along sides of spine, working up to occiput (base of head).

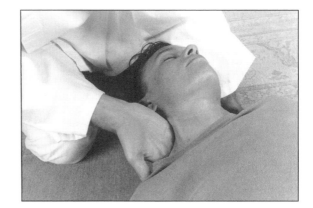

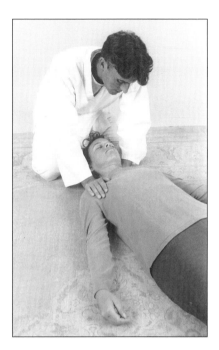

✧ *Bring your side-to-side motion to a gentle stop. Slide your left hand cupped under neck, just under occiput. Right hand holds right shoulder. Lean forward, stretching right shoulder footward and to the right, as you gently stretch the head in the opposite direction. Release, switch hand positions, and repeat, this time gently stretching head and left shoulder.*

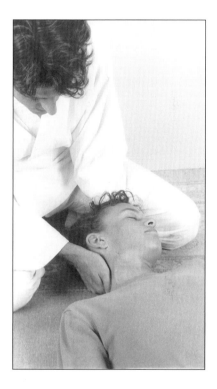

✧ *Lift head, rotate it to the left, and lower it onto your left hand and palm (fingers at base of skull, thumb around ear, back of your hand rests on floor).*

✧ *Hold right side of neck with right hand (thumb close to index finger) for 3 breaths.*

✧ *Lean forward, letting your fingertips gradually and gently carry your weight as you lean in. Hold briefly, then lean back gradually. This is called lean-hold-release. Move your fingertips down the neck a bit, **behind** the sterno-cleidomastoid muscle, and repeat the lean-hold-release motion. Continue down the side of the neck to the neck/shoulder junction.*

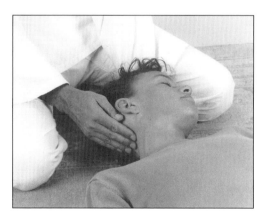

✧ *Brush firmly with side of thumb from below mastoid down neck, along shoulder and off, 3 times.*

✧ *Using your whole body, lift head very gradually, supporting your forearms on your thighs, and rotate head to center. Raise head slightly higher, then lower it as you rotate it to the right, and continue lowering it to the floor, to rest on your right palm.*

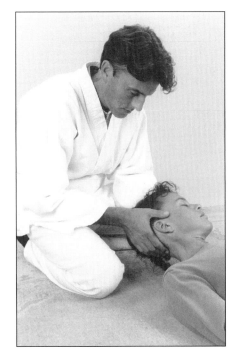

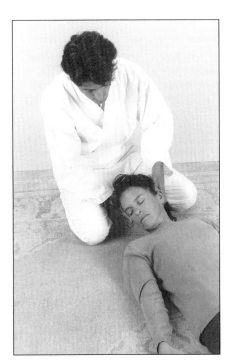

✧ *Repeat lean-hold-release and brushing down the left side of neck.*

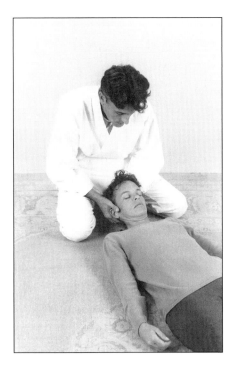

✧ *Gently raise head as before, and rotate back to center.*

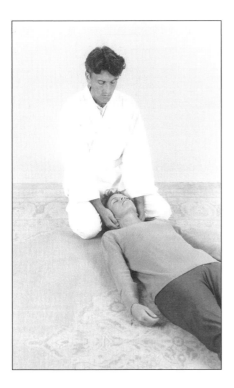

✧ *Lower head to floor, then, with fingertips behind neck on either side of spine, stretch skyward very gently.*

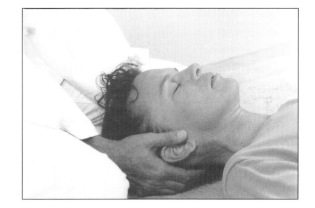

✧ *Hold sides of head around (but not covering) ears, for 3 breaths.*

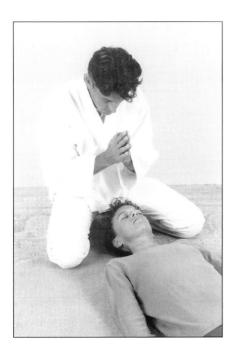

✧ *Release and bow.*

Practicing Breema

One first understands Breema through the body. That's why it's important to practice at least several times a week, because your body has to get the "taste" of Breema. Gradually you become familiar with it; body moving naturally, mind receptively attentive, and feelings supportive and present. As this taste grows, you more often allow your body to respond to the various energies it receives from people, food, the environment, and all of its interactions with the events of daily life.

When the mind is receptive rather than critical, when the feelings are supportive rather than reactive, the body manifests, using its instinctive, commonsense wisdom to balance the different energies it constantly receives.

Through connection to the body, we become present and available to life. Our feelings become interested in remaining present as we practice Breema, and through their participation, we experience a greater sense of aliveness and openness.

These definite experiences can spark a desire in us for understanding ourselves. That desire, when it is alive, creates a level of interest and receptivity in the mind that allows it to function in a new way. As we gain experience of the mind, feelings, and body working together, we become clear and organized and capable of receiving insights. These insights nurture our essence. When our essence grows, we have the possibility to become interested in self-understanding.

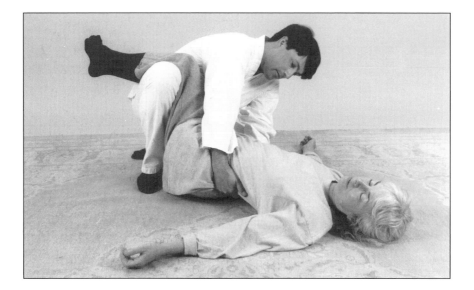

Appendices

BODY-CENTERED
MEDITATION

SELF-BREEMA

BREEMA CERTIFICATION

THE BREEMA CENTER

THE BREEMA CLINIC

EUROPEAN PROGRAMS

Body-Centered Meditation:
Having Presence and Being Present

Breema classes begin with a brief body-oriented meditation. As the students sit together with the instructor in a circle on the floor, they are guided through a series of steps that support them to become present by experiencing their body. Meditation is a way to prepare ourselves for activity, by connecting us to the principles and atmosphere we wish to carry into our day. Our meditation needs to stay connected to our purpose. Meditation is the practice of having presence and being present. The body has five "levels" or aspects.* One level is the physical body, in its natural, unmanipulated state. "Within" this body there is a deeper level, called our *essential body*. "Within" that is our *supreme* body. Our physical body is itself contained within a larger "body," consisting of the people who comprise our immediate circle, our family, friends, and community. That body is a part of a larger "body," which is comprised of all existing life.

The aim of meditation is to first come from the imaginary, conceptual world of the mind, and connect to our actual physical body. From there, we wish to go deeper, connecting to our *essential* body. When our meditation reaches this level, it influences our "outer" body, which is our circle of friends, family, and acquaintances.

If we can go deeper and connect to our *supreme body*, our meditation affects and connects us to our "outermost" body, which is all life in Existence.

This five-body schematic also shows us the relationship between our inner world and outer world. Connection to the body is the key to harmonizing our inner and outer worlds, because our physical body, our "soil body" is the bridge over which communication between our other four bodies passes.

This conceptual framework enables us to take a deeper look at the effects of meditation, but different levels, and "inner" and "outer" don't really exist as such. There is only one Existence, one Awareness, one Consciousness, one energy.

Body-Centered Meditation

❦ Find a comfortable sitting position.

❦ Close your eyes.

❦ Take a few deep breaths.

❦ Allow your shoulders to relax.

❦ As you sit, experience that the body has weight and is breathing.

❦ Let your body have a slight side-to-side rocking motion.

❦ Experience the weight of the body shifting with your movement.

❦ Slowly bring the rocking motion to a stop.

❦ Experience the effect of inhalation on the abdomen and the upper half of the body.

❦ Continue for several breaths.

❦ Experience the effect of exhalation on the abdomen and the lower half of the body.

❦ Continue for several breaths.

❦ Now, experience the effect of both inhalation and exhalation on the whole body.

❦ Slowly open your eyes, without focusing on anything for a few seconds.

You don't need Breema in order to exist.
In fact, when you know *you exist,*
you understand the true meaning of Breema,
without being identified with the name.
This Teaching is Universal.
It doesn't belong to any person or group.
Everyone who makes a direct *connection*
to their own existence "arrives" at the same place.

Self-Breema

Self-Breema exercises are treatments done on one's own body. They are an opportunity to experience being both the practitioner and the recipient at the same time.

It is possible for our body to move in accordance with natural laws, and so receive certain types of energy it needs. This is the aim of Self-Breema.

As we are, our movements are mechanical. We picked them up unconsciously from others, and they became our physical crystallizations — a very limited set of movements our body uses to do everything. We unconsciously fall back on the same postures, gestures, movements, and facial expressions we picked up, over and over again. As we go through our lives using our crystallized movements, we don't need to be fully present. We just move "on automatic."

Self-Breema first asks us to *experience* this body moving. The extra energy that we bring to *experience* our movement is the first step towards eventually being able to move with our own essential, natural movement.

Self-Breema is based on a deep understanding of the balance needed to keep movement from being too routine or too stimulating. Its movements bypass the mind, enabling us to move naturally.

When we do Self-Breema in order to help ourselves be more present and to learn to participate in the movements with our whole body, our desire for life is nurtured.

Self-Breema exercises are also a great support and preparation for practicing Breema. *Touching the Mountain: The Self-Breema Handbook — Ancient Exercises for the Modern World* is highly recommended both as a practical guide and a source of more information about this important part of the Breema method.

Breema Certification

In order to practice Breema, you will need to become a certified practitioner. The Breema Center offers a 165-hour Practitioner Certificate in Breema bodywork. The required hours consist of a series of classes which lead to proficiency in a wide variety of sequences and Self-Breema exercises, along with a thorough knowledge of the basic principles. The Certificate Program takes a minimum of six months to complete, although most students prefer to allow a year. Each student accumulates hours at his or her own pace through a combination of immersive intensive programs, weekend workshops, and weekly classes. Through this practical, holistic approach, Certified Practitioners learn to do real Breema, both in form and in their active application of the Breema principles.

The Breema Center also certifies Breema instructors. Certified Instructors have completed the Instructor Training Program which includes study with Dr. Jon Schreiber, the Director, and senior faculty instructors at the Breema Center. Certified Instructors have had, at minimum, several years of practicing Breema and have received intensive training in presenting Breema. Instructors are re-certified yearly.

The Breema Center

The Breema Center was founded in Berkeley, California in 1980 to introduce Breema to the Western world, and is currently directed by Dr. Jon Schreiber. Students are given a thorough training in the movements, sequences, principles, and Self-Breema exercises that comprise the Breema method. Emphasis is placed on learning with the whole body, Breema as an ongoing practice, and on the integration of the principles in daily life. The Center offers a variety of formats, including weekday and evening classes, weekend workshops, and intensives from one to three weeks long.

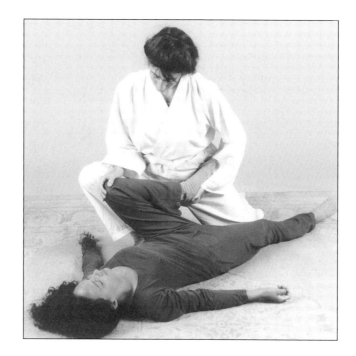

The Breema Center is the world training headquarters for Breema, and offers a Certification Program for practitioners, instructor training and certification, and continuing education. The Center is actively involved in creating comprehensive archives, and in the publication of informational and educational media. Breema classes taught by Certified Breema Instructors are available in many cities in the United States, as well as in Europe, British Columbia, Mexico, and Israel. The Breema Center maintains a directory of Certified Practitioners and Certified Instructors. This information is available on the Internet at our Web site, or you may call us to request a copy.

The Breema Center
6076 Claremont Avenue
Oakland, CA 94618
510-428-0937
e-mail: center@breema.com
Web site: http://www.breema.com

The Advanced Arts Breema Chiropractic Clinic

We have been using Breema bodywork, Self-Breema exercises, and the principles of Breema since 1981 to help revitalize patients with acute and chronic conditions. Nearly everyone experiences a diminution of symptoms, and many reach a level of health that surpasses their pre-illness or pre-injury status. Our patients share with us a profound gratitude for the improvement in health, increase in flexibility, and greater sense of well-being, harmony, and interest in life that come with practicing and receiving Breema.

We have found Breema a phenomenal catalyst for the body's self-healing processes, yet also so safe, so natural, and so respectful of the body that it is an ideal form of complementary therapy for infants, children, pregnant women, and the elderly, as well as for people with conditions which require precise and delicate treatment.

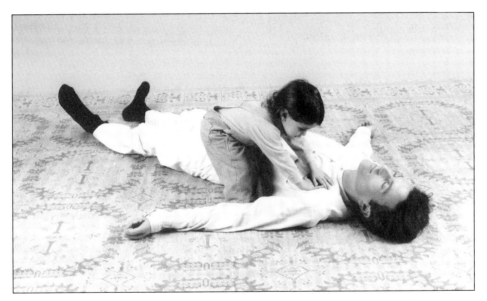

Sarita, Dr. Schreiber's two-year-old daughter, already enjoys Breema's playful movements.

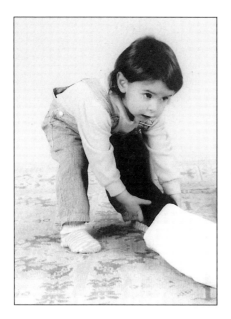

There is no doubt that the increasing challenges to health presented by modern life will be accompanied by the discovery of many more therapeutic applications of Breema. We hope to provide an ever-increasing number of people the opportunity to experience the physical, mental, and emotional benefits of Breema, as well as its support in understanding the laws that offer us a means of living an essential, harmonious life.

— Jon Schreiber, D.C.,
and the Advanced Arts Breema staff

Advanced Arts Breema Chiropractic Clinic
6201 Florio Street
Oakland, California 94618
510-428-1234
fax: 510-428-2705
Web site: http://www.breema.com

European Training Programs

The Breema Center conducts European Practitioner Certification Programs, which are currently based in Austria and Germany. The European programs are directed by Pari Schneider and Aron Saltiel.

Pari Schneider has been practicing Breema for over eleven years, and teaching extensively for nine. He studied for many years with Malichek Mooshan at the Breema Center. Mr. Schneider also trained with Dr. Schreiber at Advanced Arts Breema Chiropractic Clinic. In addition to directing the German Certification Program, Mr. Schneider teaches classes and workshops throughout Europe. His clear presentation and deep connection with Breema have inspired many people to become committed students of this unique system.

Aron Saltiel was introduced to Breema over fifteen years ago. He organized the first seminars in Europe, and then returned to the U.S. to complete his instructor certification at the Breema Center. He and his wife, Claudia Saltiel, have trained extensively with the Center's Director, and with Pari Schneider. Claudia Saltiel has taught in a variety of settings, including workshops for teachers and others in health and social service professions. Aron Saltiel is a clinical psychologist in practice in Graz, Austria. He uses Breema in his clinical practice, and organizes training programs for psychotherapists throughout Europe. Mr. Saltiel directs the Austrian Certification Program.

In addition to maintaining their active teaching schedules, Mr. Schneider and Mr. Saltiel organize translation of written material about Breema.

For additional information:

Pari Schneider
Panoramastr. 19
D-77815 Bühl b. Baden
Germany

phone: 49-7223250460
fax: 49-7223250181

Aron and Claudia Saltiel
Heinrichstr. 131
A-8010 Graz
Austria

phone and fax: 43-316386417
e-mail: a_saltiel@mail.styria.com

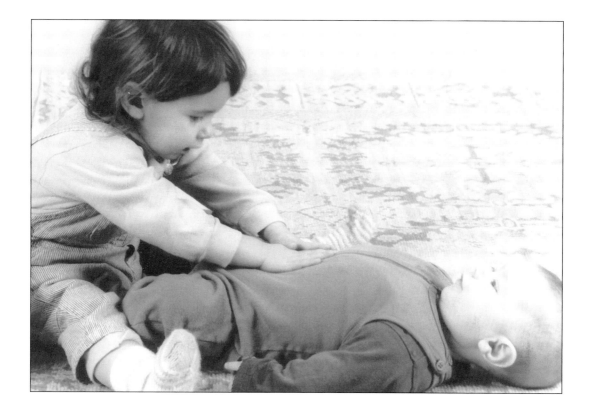

This book presents Breema for both beginners and advanced students. Stay with what feels right and makes sense to you, and let go of whatever doesn't openly speak to you. When the right time comes, you will find an inner recognition of that which is for you, that which you can apply in your daily life.

With all my Being, I wish you well. I wish you an active and healthy existence in your body.